Everyday
low carb

pil

Publications International, Ltd.

Microwave Cooking: Microwave ovens vary in wattage. Use the cooking times as guidelines and check for doneness before adding more time.

Nutritional Analysis: Every effort has been made to check the accuracy of the nutritional information that appears with each recip. However, because numerous variables account for a wide range of values for certain foods, nutritive analyses in this book should be considered approximate.

Note: This publication is only intended to provide general information. The information is specifically not intended to be a substitute for medical diagnosis or treatment by your physician or other health care professional. You should always consult your own physician or other health care professionals about any medical questions, diagnosis, or treatment. (Products vary among manufacturers. Please check labels carefully to confirm nutritional values.)

Let's get social!
@Publications_International
@PublicationsInternational
www.pilbooks.com

contents

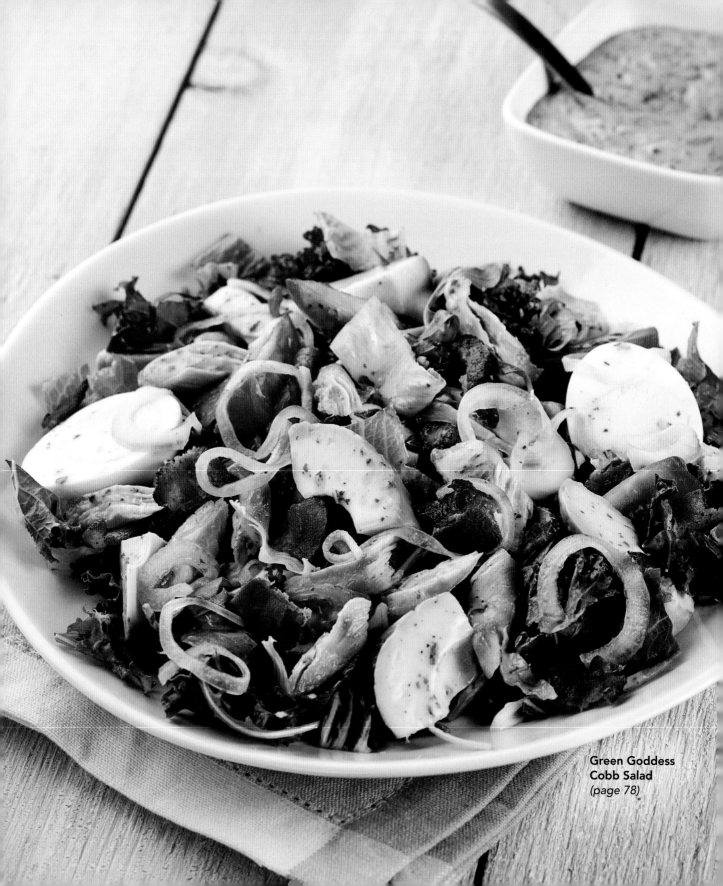

**Green Goddess
Cobb Salad**
(page 78)

introduction

WHAT IS A LOW-CARB DIET?

Just as it says—a low-carb diet restricts carbohydrates in the diet. Foods that contribute carbs are limited—grains, starchy vegetables and fruit— while foods high in protein and fat are emphasized.

Primarily, individuals are drawn to a low-carb diet to lose weight. The low-carb diet will contribute to weight loss due to its restrictive nature, but it's not as restrictive as the keto diet. Along with weight loss, the low-carb diet has shown effective results in reducing risk factors associated with type 2 diabetes, metabolic syndrome, hypertension and heart disease. So all-in-all it sounds good, right?

WHAT ARE CARBOHYDRATES?

Carbohydrates are the primary source of food our body needs for energy. Carbohydrates include simple carbohydrates (table sugar, honey) and complex carbohydrates which contain fiber (starches, fruits, vegetables and whole grains).

Carbohydrates are an important part of one's diet and are recommended as part of a well-balanced dietary intake. It's no secret that many people love to eat carbohydrates, but if eaten in excess of what is required, weight gain can occur resulting in overweight or obesity. In the case of the low-carb diet when carbohydrates are restricted, weight can be lost. Therefore, many have turned to a low-carb diet; some with impressive results.

HOW DOES THE DIET WORK?

The low-carb diet can help a person lose weight because when a carbohydrate-rich food source is replaced with higher fat and protein foods, the body needs to use fat and protein sources to provide energy. By increasing the fat-burning processes in the body, the body goes into what can be called a "dietary ketosis," where fats and protein are used for energy. And because fats and protein-rich sources of food take longer to digest in the body, one feels fuller for longer periods of time so these foods can also work as sort of an appetite depressant.

Carbohydrates are the body's preferred and primary energy source. Simple carbohydrates are digested directly into the bloodstream as blood sugar (glucose). When blood sugars increase, the body releases insulin to help the glucose enter the body's cells. Some glucose is immediately used for energy, for activities for daily living, while extra glucose is stored in the liver, muscles and other cells for later use or it may be converted to fat, if not needed right away. On the other hand, complex carbohydrates are broken down into simple sugars during digestion, where they are absorbed into the bloodstream. Complex carbohydrates take longer to digest than simple carbohydrates as they provide dietary fiber. They also help with reducing constipation and digestive concerns.

So, the thinking behind following a low-carb diet is that by reducing carbohydrates in the diet, the body will burn stored fat for energy and individuals will ultimately lose weight.

WHAT CAN I EAT ON A LOW-CARB DIET?

The low-carb diet emphasizes the consumption of high-protein foods like meat, poultry, fish and eggs, and some non-starchy vegetables while eliminating the majority of grains, legumes, fruits, breads, pastas, starchy vegetables and high-sugar foods.

A very restrictive daily limit of 20 to 60 grams of carbohydrates may be the goal but less restrictive limits of up to 150 grams of carbohydrates per day are suggested. Some diets greatly restrict carbohydrates at first, then slowly add more in as the diet progresses along. Being too restrictive can be difficult to follow particularly for any length of time.

To put it in perspective, a typical American diet can include upwards of 200 to 300 grams or more of carbohydrates per day, as noted in the recommendations of the Dietary Guidelines for Americans. Recommendations indicate that carbohydrates should comprise 45 to 65 percent of your total daily calorie intake.

HOW QUICKLY WILL RESULTS OCCUR?

When following very restrictive low-carb diets, one may see short-term weight loss quickly. This can sometimes be a motivator to keep going. But, unless the diet is maintained, the weight loss will likely resume once carbohydrates are re-entered in the diet.

ARE THERE ANY RISKS TO A LOW-CARB DIET?

It's important to check with your doctor before starting any restrictive diet. Your doctor can assess your health status to determine if you have any conditions that can be affected with this or any type of weight-loss diet. But note, other conditions such as constipation, dehydration, headaches, weakness, fatigue, muscle aches and/or even bad breath are possible when restricting certain nutrients from your diet. Long-term effects could even be greater with possible bone loss or other chronic conditions.

BE SMART...EDUCATE YOURSELF

Before following any diet, take the time to educate yourself on the diet, what you can eat and what foods are restricted. Short term, many weight loss diets will not be harmful and people receive the positive results they are seeking. But in the long term, it's important to consult with professionals as a doctor or registered dietitian nutritionist. They can be sure to steer you in the right direction.

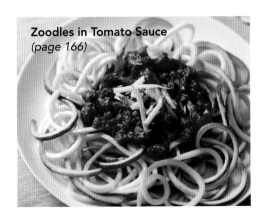

Zoodles in Tomato Sauce
(page 166)

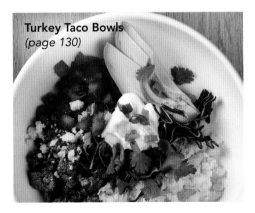

Turkey Taco Bowls
(page 130)

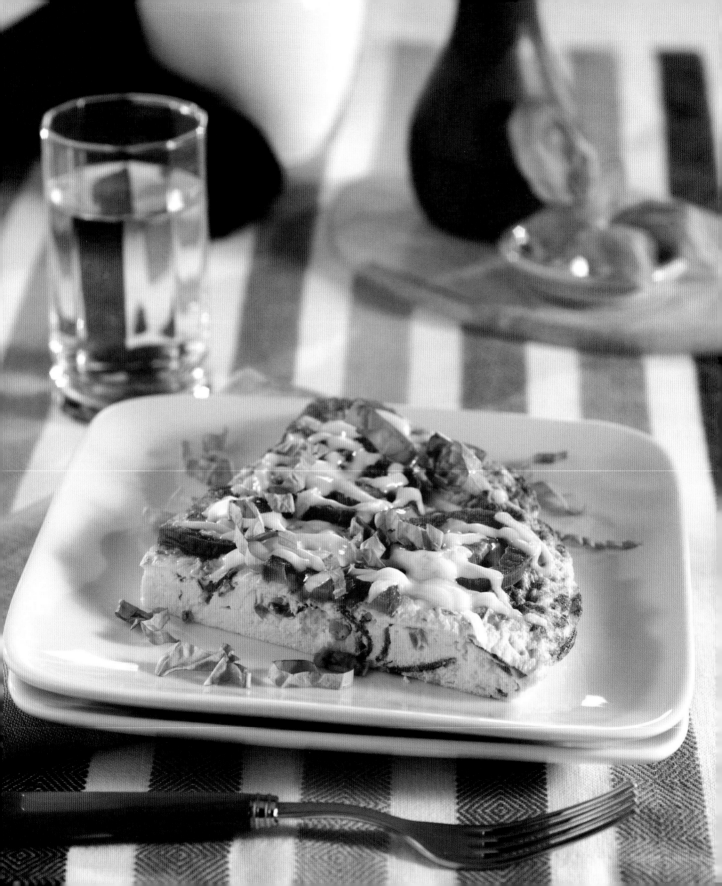

brunch

Pepperoni Frittata

Makes 4 servings

2 cups egg substitute

⅓ cup fat-free evaporated milk

1 ounce turkey pepperoni slices, chopped (about 16 slices)

¼ cup finely chopped green onions

½ teaspoon dried rosemary

½ teaspoon dried basil

⅛ teaspoon salt

⅛ teaspoon black pepper

2 medium plum tomatoes, thinly sliced

¾ cup (3 ounces) shredded mozzarella cheese

Fresh basil leaves, cut into thin strips (optional)

1. Preheat broiler.

2. Combine egg substitute, milk, pepperoni, green onions, rosemary, basil, salt and pepper in medium bowl.

3. Spray 10-inch nonstick skillet with nonstick cooking spray; heat over medium heat. Add egg mixture; reduce heat to medium-low. Cook 8 to 10 minutes or until edge is set (center will still be wet).

4. Place skillet under broiler 4 inches away from heat source; broil 1 minute or until eggs are set.

5. Arrange tomatoes on top of frittata; sprinkle with cheese. Broil 1 minute or until cheese is melted. Let stand 5 minutes before serving. Garnish with basil.

Ham and Vegetable Omelet

Makes 4 servings

PER SERVING

126 **calories**
4g **total fat**
8g **carbs**
7g **net carbs**
1g **dietary fiber**
16g **protein**

2 ounces diced 95% fat-free ham (about ½ cup)

1 small onion, diced

½ medium green bell pepper, diced

½ medium red bell pepper, diced

2 cloves garlic, minced

1½ cups cholesterol-free egg substitute *or* 6 eggs, beaten

⅛ teaspoon black pepper

½ cup (2 ounces) shredded reduced-fat Colby cheese, divided

1 medium tomato, chopped

Hot pepper sauce (optional)

1. Spray 12-inch nonstick skillet with nonstick cooking spray; heat over medium-high heat. Add ham, onion, bell peppers and garlic; cook and stir 5 minutes or until vegetables are crisp-tender. Transfer mixture to large bowl.

2. Wipe out skillet with paper towels; spray with cooking spray. Heat over medium-high heat. Pour egg substitute into skillet; sprinkle with black pepper. Cook 2 minutes or until bottom is set, lifting edge of egg with spatula to allow uncooked portion to flow underneath. Reduce heat to medium-low; cover and cook 4 minutes or until top is set.

3. Gently slide omelet onto large serving plate; spoon ham mixture down center. Sprinkle with ¼ cup cheese. Carefully fold two sides of omelet over ham mixture; sprinkle with remaining ¼ cup cheese and tomato. Cut into four wedges; serve immediately with hot pepper sauce, if desired.

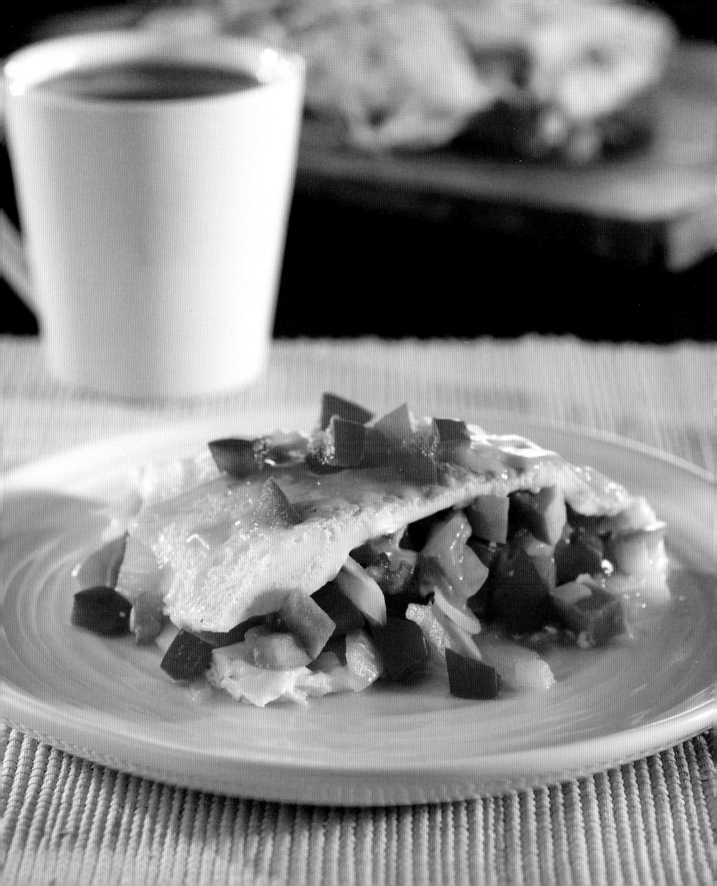

Asparagus Frittata Prosciutto Cups

Makes 12 cups (6 servings)

 1   tablespoon olive oil

 1   small red onion, finely chopped

1½   cups sliced asparagus (½-inch pieces)

 1   clove garlic, minced

12   thin slices prosciutto

 8   eggs

 ½   cup (2 ounces) grated white Cheddar cheese

 ¼   cup grated Parmesan cheese

 2   tablespoons whipping cream

 ⅛   teaspoon black pepper

1. Preheat oven to 375°F. Spray 12 standard (2½-inch) muffin cups with nonstick cooking spray.

2. Heat oil in large skillet over medium heat. Add onion; cook and stir 4 minutes or until softened. Add asparagus and garlic; cook and stir 8 minutes or until asparagus is crisp-tender. Set aside to cool slightly.

3. Line each prepared muffin cup with prosciutto slice. (Prosciutto should cover cup as much as possible, with edges extending above muffin pan.) Whisk eggs, Cheddar and Parmesan cheeses, cream and pepper in large bowl until well blended. Stir in asparagus mixture until blended. Pour into prosciutto-lined cups, filling about three-fourths full.

4. Bake about 20 minutes or until frittatas are puffed and golden brown and edges are pulling away from pan. Cool in pan 10 minutes. Remove to wire rack; serve warm or at room temperature.

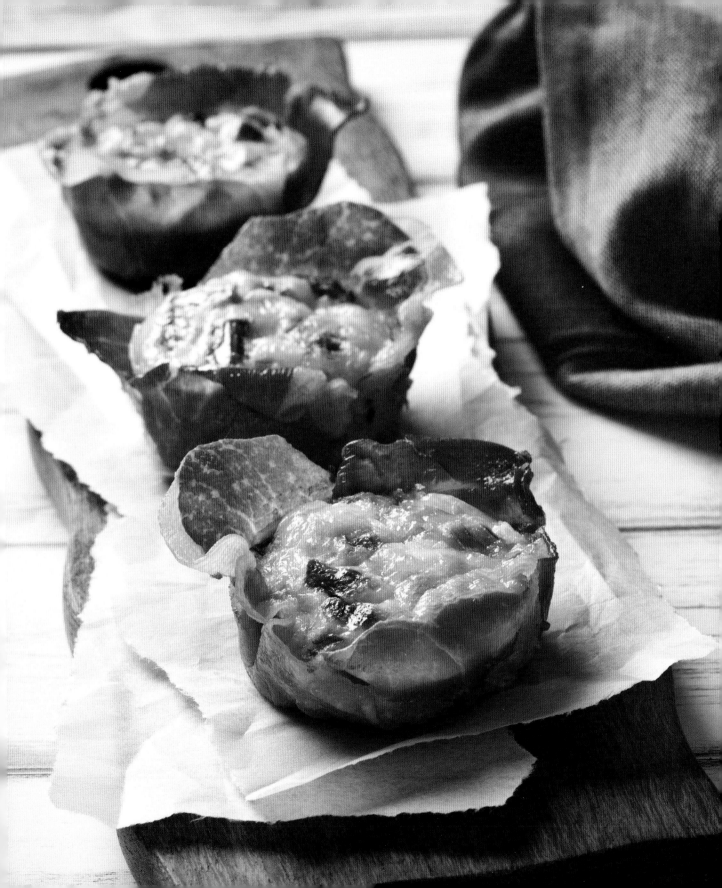

Crustless Ham and Asparagus Quiche

Makes 6 servings

- 2 **cups sliced asparagus (½-inch pieces)**
- 1 **red bell pepper, chopped**
- 1 **tablespoon water**
- 1 **cup whole milk**
- 4 **eggs**
- 4 **ounces chopped deli ham**
- 2 **tablespoons chopped fresh tarragon or basil**
- ½ **teaspoon salt**
- ¼ **teaspoon black pepper**
- ½ **cup (2 ounces) finely shredded Swiss cheese**

1. Preheat oven to 350°F. Combine asparagus, bell pepper and water in microwavable bowl. Cover with waxed paper; microwave on HIGH 2 minutes or until vegetables are crisp-tender. Drain vegetables.

2. Whisk milk and eggs in large bowl until well blended. Stir in vegetables, ham, tarragon, salt and black pepper. Pour into 9-inch pie plate.

3. Bake 35 minutes. Sprinkle cheese over quiche; bake 5 minutes or until center is set and cheese is melted. Let stand 5 minutes before serving. Cut into six wedges.

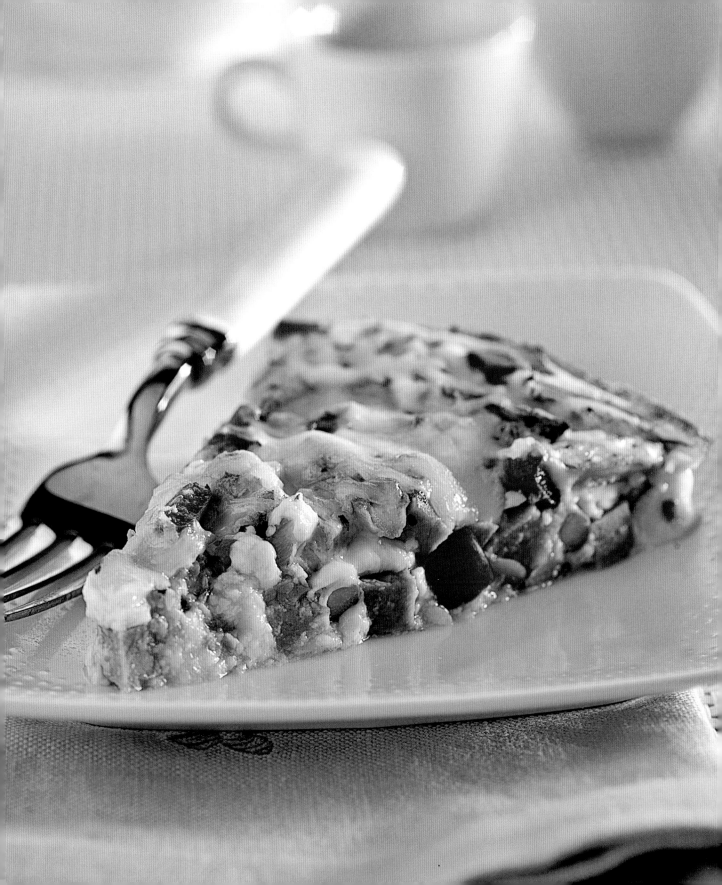

Smoked Salmon Omelet Roll-Ups

PER SERVING

100 **calories**
5g **total fat**
1g **carbs**
1g **net carbs**
0g **dietary fiber**
14g **protein**

Makes about 24 pieces (6 servings)

- **4 eggs**
- ⅛ **teaspoon black pepper**
- ¼ **cup chive and onion cream cheese, softened**
- **1 package (about 4 ounces) smoked salmon (lox), cut into bite-size pieces**

1. Beat eggs and pepper in small bowl until well blended (no streaks of white showing). Spray large nonstick skillet with nonstick cooking spray; heat over medium-high heat.

2. Pour half of egg mixture into skillet; tilt skillet to completely coat bottom with thin layer of eggs. Cook, without stirring, 2 to 4 minutes or until eggs are set. Use spatula to carefully loosen omelet from skillet; slide onto cutting board. Repeat with remaining egg mixture to make second omelet.

3. Spread 2 tablespoons cream cheese over each omelet; top with smoked salmon pieces. Roll up omelets tightly; wrap in plastic wrap and refrigerate at least 30 minutes. Cut off ends, then cut rolls crosswise into ½-inch slices.

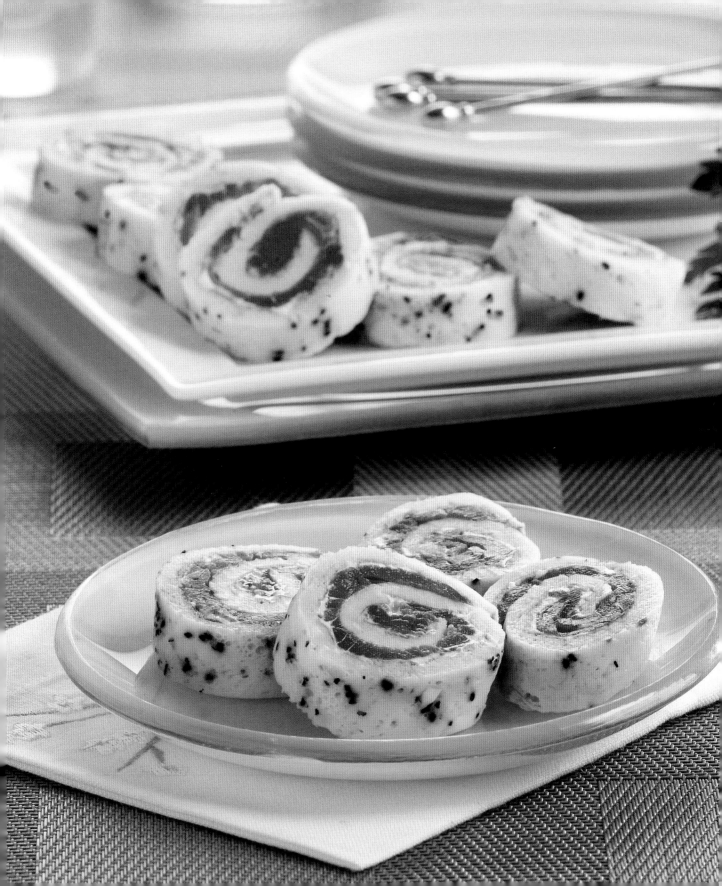

Bacon-Kale Quiche

Makes 8 servings

Crust

- ¾ cup coconut flour
- ¾ cup almond flour
- ¼ teaspoon salt
- 2 eggs
- 6 tablespoons coconut oil or butter, melted

Filling

- 8 eggs
- ½ cup whipping cream
- 1 package (12 ounces) bacon
- 1 cup chopped onion
- 3 cups tightly packed chopped stemmed kale
- ½ cup finely shredded Parmesan cheese
- ¼ cup finely chopped sun-dried tomatoes

1. Preheat oven to 375°F. Combine coconut flour, almond flour and salt in medium bowl. Stir in 2 eggs and coconut oil until well blended. Press onto bottom and up side of deep-dish pie plate. Bake 5 minutes.

2. Whisk eggs and cream in large bowl until well blended. Cook bacon in large skillet until crisp. Drain on paper towels; chop when cool enough to handle. Add onion and kale to drippings in skillet; cook and stir over medium heat about 5 minutes or until onion is golden and kale is wilted. Add vegetables and drippings to eggs; mix well. Stir in Parmesan cheese, tomatoes and bacon. Pour into prepared crust.

3. Bake 40 minutes or until quiche is puffed and knife inserted into center comes out clean, covering edges of crust with foil after 20 minutes to prevent overbrowning. Let stand 20 minutes before cutting.

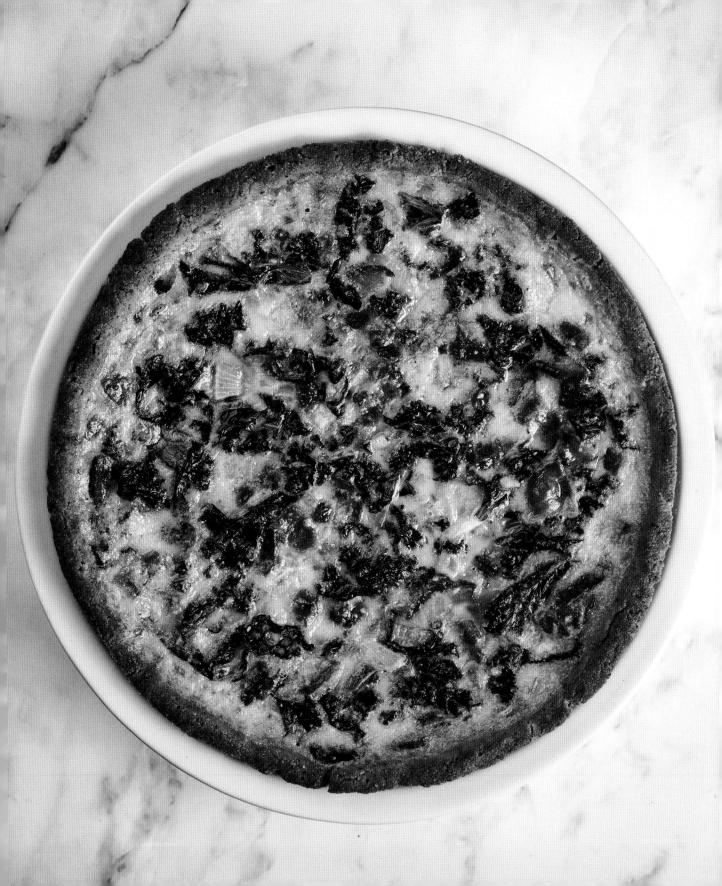

Cheese Soufflé

Makes 4 servings

¼ cup (½ stick) butter

¼ cup almond flour

1½ cups milk, warmed to room temperature

¼ teaspoon salt

¼ teaspoon ground red pepper

⅛ teaspoon black pepper

6 eggs, separated

1 cup (4 ounces) shredded Cheddar cheese

Pinch cream of tartar (optional)

1. Preheat oven to 375°F. Grease four 2-cup soufflé dishes or one 2-quart soufflé dish.

2. Melt butter in large saucepan over medium-low heat. Add almond flour; whisk 2 minutes or until mixture just begins to color. Gradually whisk in milk. Add salt, red pepper and black pepper; whisk until mixture comes to a boil and thickens. Remove from heat. Stir in egg yolks, one at a time, and cheese.

3. Beat egg whites and cream of tartar in large bowl with electric mixer at high speed until stiff peaks form.

4. Gently fold egg whites into cheese mixture until almost combined. (Some streaks of white should remain.) Transfer mixture to prepared dishes.

5. Bake small soufflés about 20 minutes (30 to 40 minutes for large soufflé) or until puffed and browned and tester inserted into center comes out moist but clean. Serve immediately.

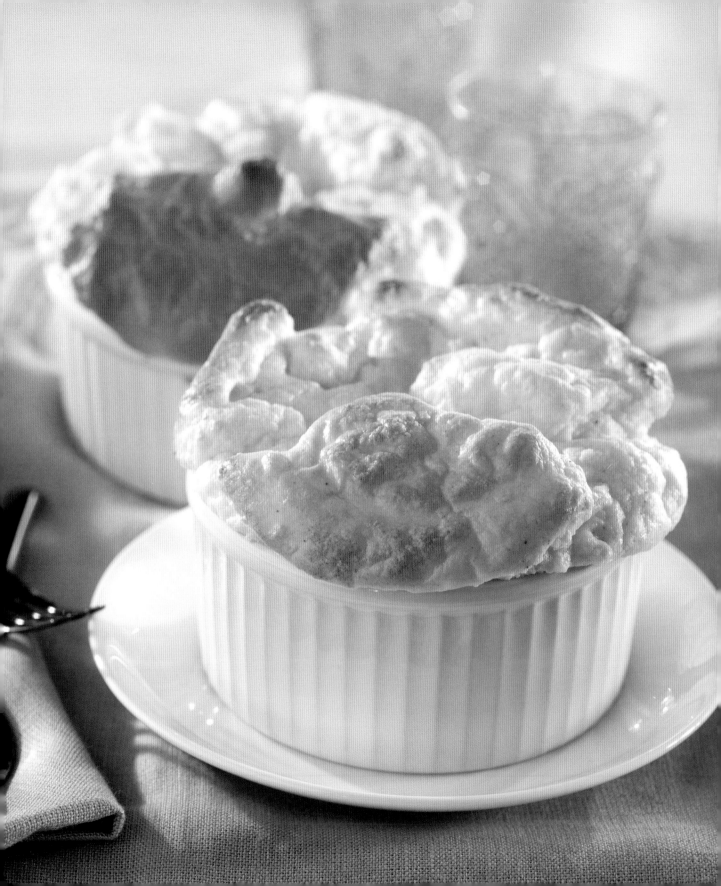

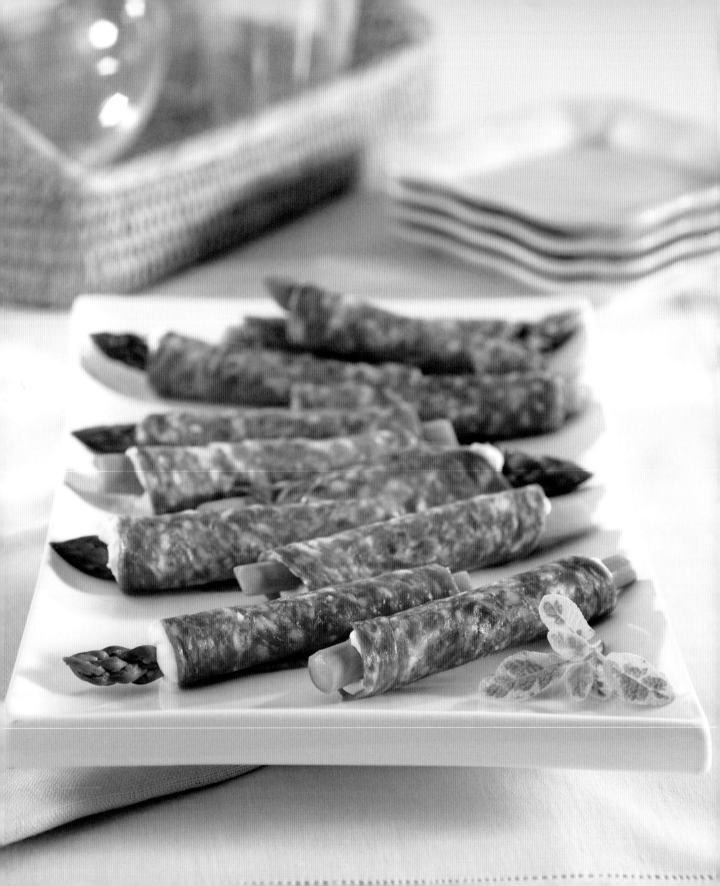

appetizers

PER SERVING

40 calories
3g **total fat**
1g **carbs**
1g **net carbs**
0g **dietary fiber**
2g **protein**

Asparagus Roll-Ups

Makes about 24 roll-ups

1 **pound asparagus, tough ends trimmed (about 24 spears)**

½ **(8-ounce) package cream cheese, softened**

½ **pound thinly sliced salami**

1. Cut asparagus into lengths 1 inch longer than width of salami. Reserve bottoms for another use. Simmer asparagus in salted water in large skillet 4 to 5 minutes or until crisp-tender. Drain; immediately immerse in cold water to stop the cooking process. Drain; pat dry with paper towel.

2. Spread about 1 teaspoon cream cheese evenly over one side of each salami slice. Roll up 1 asparagus spear with each salami slice.

3. Cover and refrigerate. Let stand at room temperature 10 minutes before serving.

Roasted Red Pepper Dip

Makes 8 servings

PER SERVING

140 calories
11g **total fat**
3g **carbs**
3g **net carbs**
0g **dietary fiber**
5g **protein**

2 cups crumbled feta cheese

2 tablespoons garlic-flavored olive oil

¼ teaspoon black pepper

1 jar (12 ounces) roasted red peppers, drained

Cut-up fresh vegetables

1. Process cheese, oil and black pepper in food processor 1 minute or until smooth.

2. Add red peppers. Process 10 to 15 seconds or until mixed but not puréed. Serve with vegetables.

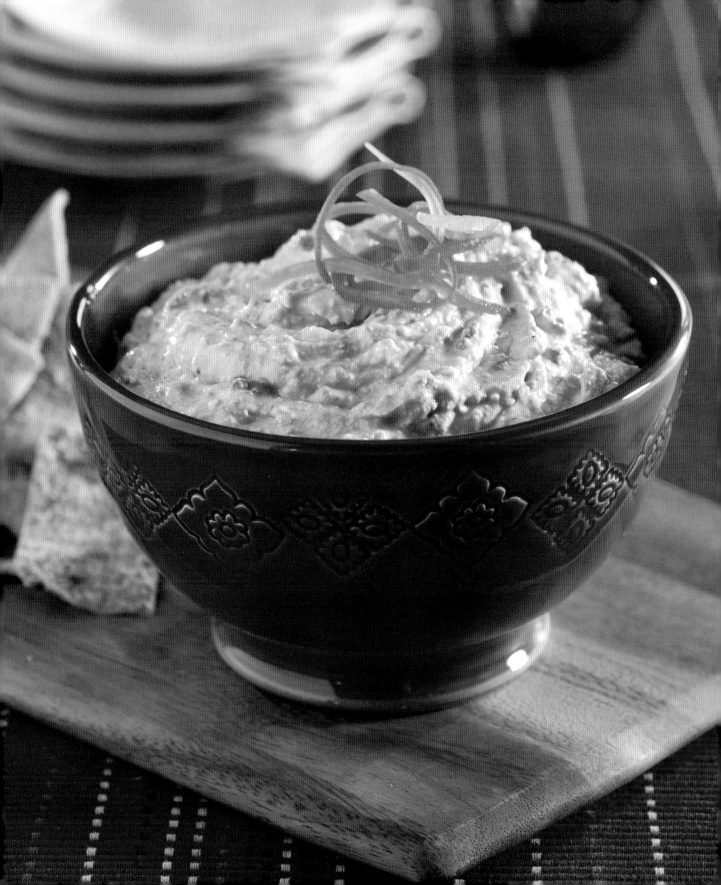

Spinach, Artichoke and Feta Dip

Makes about 1½ cups (about 6 servings)

PER SERVING

100 **calories**
7g **total fat**
6g **carbs**
5g **net carbs**
1g **dietary fiber**
5g **protein**

- ½ **cup thawed frozen chopped spinach**
- 1 **cup crumbled feta cheese**
- ½ **teaspoon black pepper**
- 1 **cup marinated artichokes, undrained**
- **Pita chips and/or cucumber slices**

1. Place spinach in small microwavable bowl; microwave on HIGH 2 minutes.

2. Place cheese and pepper in food processor. Process 1 minute or until finely chopped. Add artichokes and spinach; process 30 seconds until well mixed but not puréed. Serve with pita chips and/or cucumber slices.

Note: To keep your carb count down, limit the number of pita chips consumed.

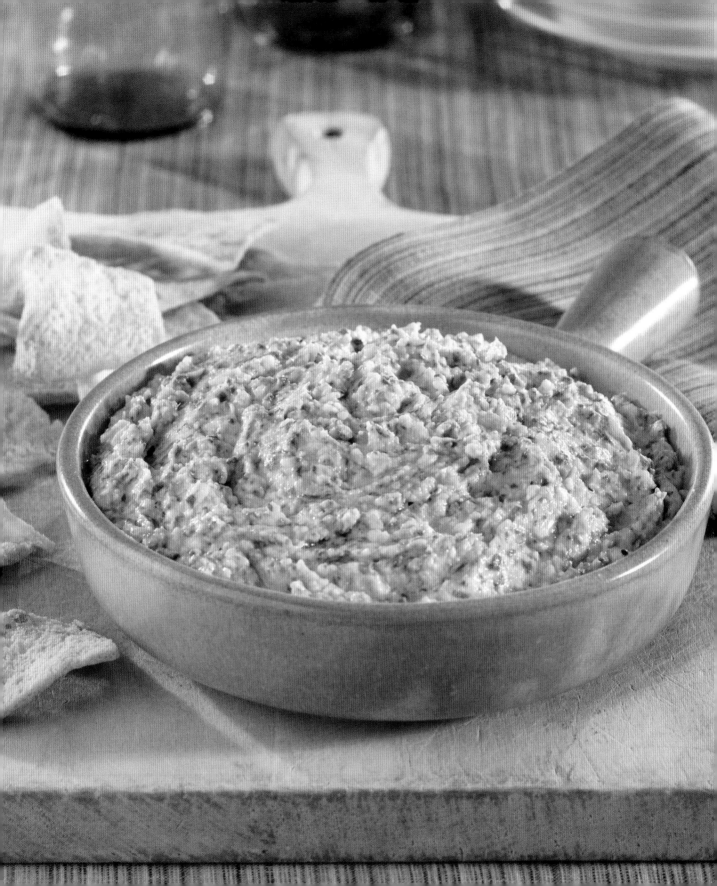

Kale Chips

Makes 6 servings

- 1 **large bunch kale (about 1 pound)**
- 1 **to 2 tablespoons olive oil**
- 1 **teaspoon garlic salt or other seasoned salt**

1. Preheat oven to 350°F. Line baking sheets with parchment paper.

2. Wash kale and pat dry with paper towels. Remove center ribs and stems; discard. Cut leaves into 2- to 3-inch-wide pieces.

3. Combine leaves, oil and garlic salt in large bowl; toss to coat. Spread onto prepared baking sheets.

4. Bake 10 to 15 minutes or until edges are lightly browned and leaves are crisp.* Cool completely on baking sheets. Store in airtight container.

If the leaves are lightly browned but not crisp, turn oven off and let chips stand in oven until crisp, about 10 minutes. Do not keep the oven on as the chips will burn easily.

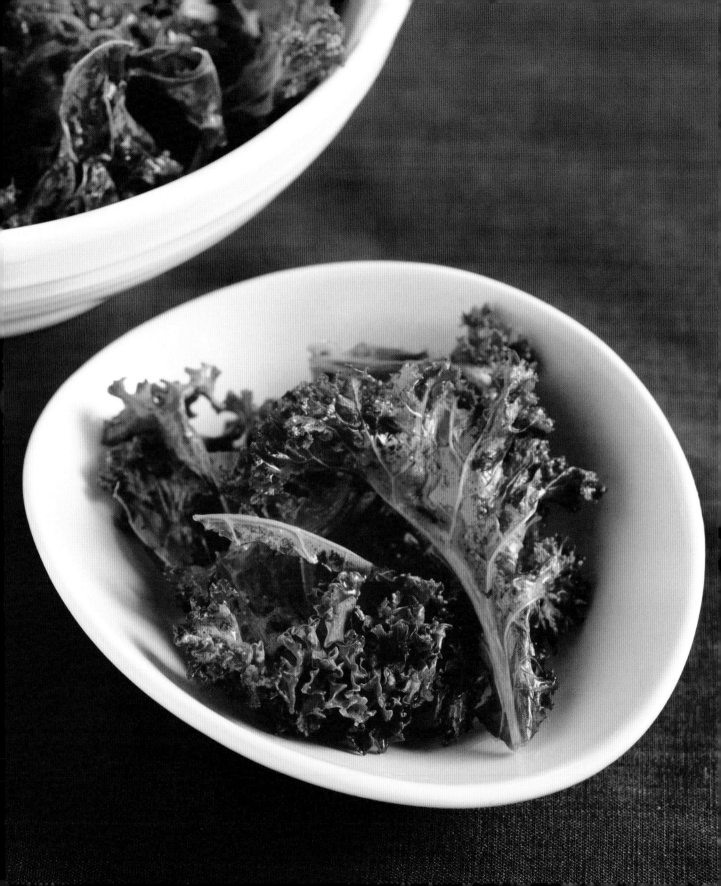

Creamy Cashew Spread

Makes about ½ cup (6 servings)

1   cup raw cashew nuts

2   tablespoons lemon juice

1   tablespoon tahini

½   teaspoon salt

½   teaspoon black pepper

2   teaspoons minced fresh herbs, such as basil, parsley or oregano (optional)

Assorted bread toasts and/or vegetable slices

1. Rinse cashews and place in medium bowl. Cover with water by at least 2 inches. Soak 4 hours or overnight. Drain cashews, reserving soaking water.

2. Place cashews, 2 tablespoons reserved water, lemon juice, tahini, salt and pepper in food processor or blender; process several minutes or until smooth. Add additional water, 1 tablespoon at a time, until desired consistency is reached.

3. Cover and refrigerate until ready to serve. Stir in herbs, if desired, just before serving. Serve with assorted bread toasts and/or vegetable slices.

Tip: Use this dip as a spread for sandwiches or as a pasta topping. Thin it with additional liquid as needed. You can also use it in place of sour cream as a topping for tacos and chili.

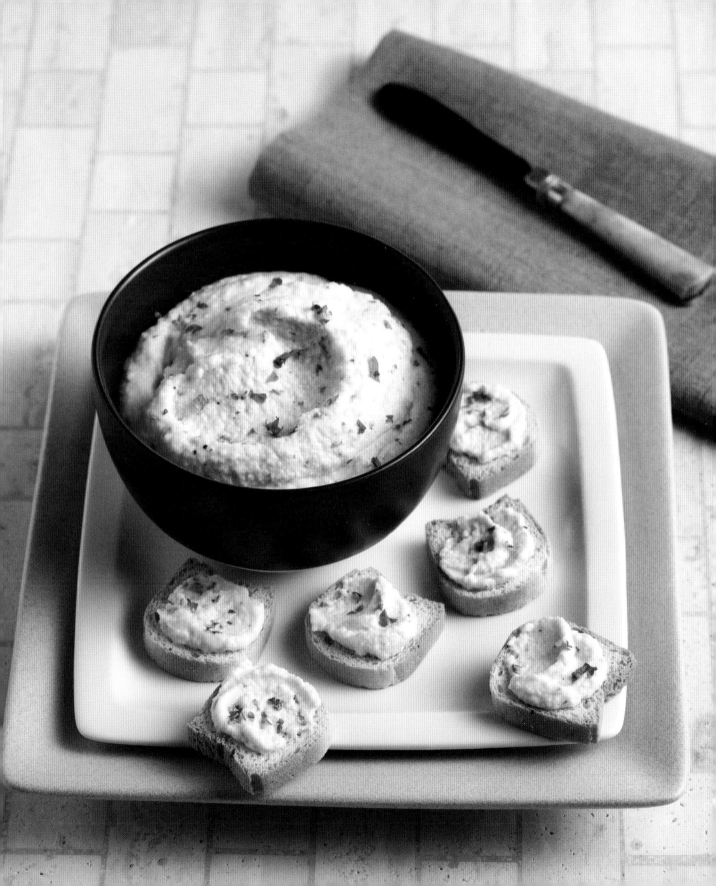

Swimming Tuna Dip

Makes 6 servings

1 cup low-fat (1%) cottage cheese

1 tablespoon reduced-fat mayonnaise

1 tablespoon lemon juice

2 teaspoons dry ranch-style salad dressing mix

1 can (5 ounces) chunk white tuna packed in water, drained and flaked

2 tablespoons sliced green onion or chopped celery

1 teaspoon dried parsley flakes

1 package (12 ounces) peeled baby carrots

1. Combine cottage cheese, mayonnaise, lemon juice and salad dressing mix in food processor or blender. Cover and blend until smooth.

2. Combine tuna, green onion and parsley flakes in small bowl. Stir in cottage cheese mixture. Serve with carrots.

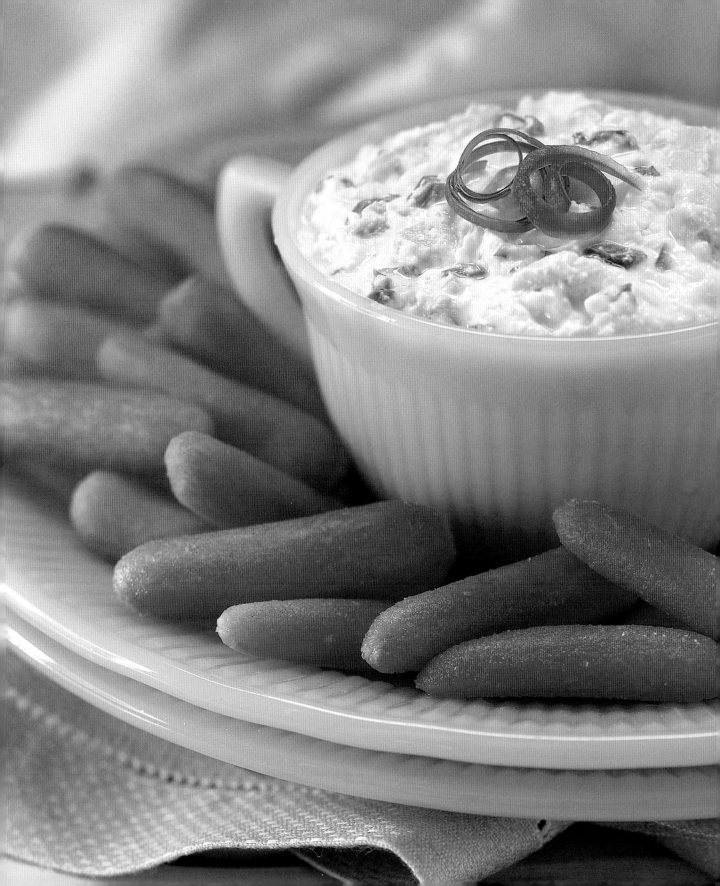

PER SERVING

210 calories
19g **total fat**
5g **carbs**
4g **net carbs**
1g **dietary fiber**
9g **protein**

Taco Dip

Makes 10 servings

12 ounces cream cheese, softened

½ cup sour cream

2 teaspoons chili powder

1½ teaspoons ground cumin

⅛ teaspoon ground red pepper

½ cup salsa

1 cup (4 ounces) shredded Cheddar cheese

1 cup (4 ounces) shredded Monterey Jack cheese

½ cup diced plum tomatoes

⅓ cup sliced green onions

¼ cup sliced pitted black olives

¼ cup sliced pimiento-stuffed green olives

Shredded lettuce

Tortilla chips and blue corn chips

1. Combine cream cheese, sour cream, chili powder, cumin and red pepper in large bowl; mix until well blended. Stir in salsa.

2. Spread dip onto serving platter. Top with cheeses, tomatoes, green onions and olives. Sprinkle shredded lettuce around edges of dip.

3. Serve with tortilla chips and blue corn chips.

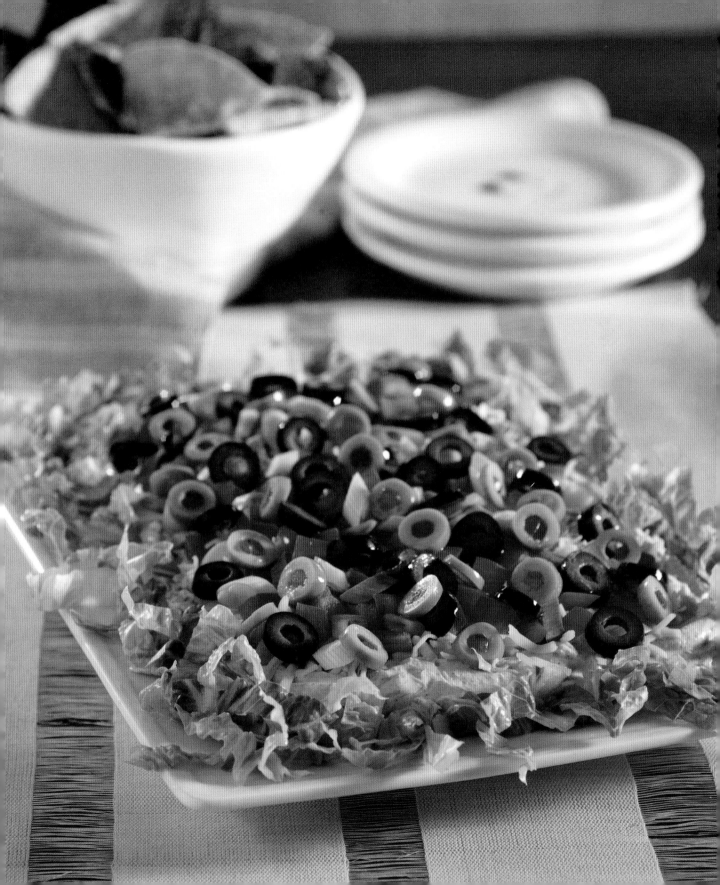

Mini Marinated Beef Skewers

Makes 18 appetizers

PER SERVING

45 **calories**
2g **total fat**
1g **carbs**
1g **net carbs**
0g **dietary fiber**
5g **protein**

1 boneless beef top sirloin
   (about 1 pound)

2 tablespoons dry sherry

2 tablespoons soy sauce

1 tablespoon dark sesame oil

2 cloves garlic, minced

18 cherry tomatoes

Lettuce leaves (optional)

1. Cut beef crosswise into ⅛-inch slices. Place in large resealable food storage bag. Combine sherry, soy sauce, sesame oil and garlic in small bowl; pour over beef. Seal bag; turn to coat. Marinate in refrigerator at least 30 minutes or up to 2 hours. Soak 18 (6-inch) wooden skewers in water 20 minutes.

2. Preheat broiler. Drain beef; discard marinade. Weave beef accordion-style onto skewers. Place on rack of broiler pan.

3. Broil 4 to 5 inches from heat 2 minutes. Turn skewers over; broil 2 minutes or until beef is barely pink in center. Place 1 cherry tomato on each skewer. Serve warm or at room temperature over lettuce leaves, if desired.

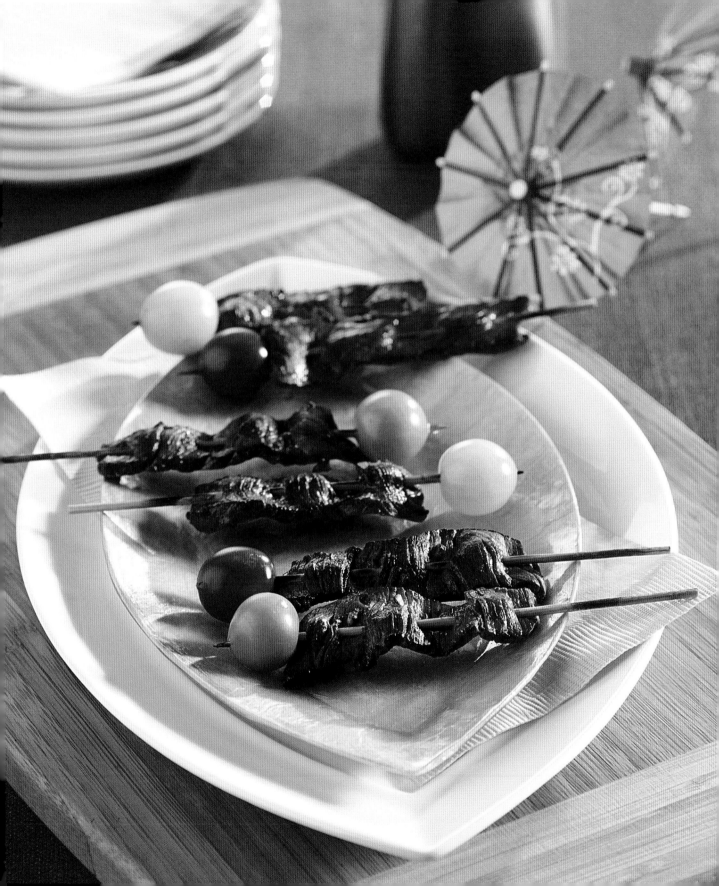

Smoked Salmon Spirals

Makes 2 servings

PER SERVING

100 **calories**
4.5g **total fat**
11g **carbs**
10g **net carbs**
1g **dietary fiber**
7g **protein**

- 2 tablespoons low-fat cream cheese
- 1 light sun-dried tomato flatbread
- 2 ounces smoked salmon (lox)
- ½ cup baby arugula
- ½ cup thinly sliced red bell pepper

Spread cream cheese on flatbread. Layer with smoked salmon, arugula and bell pepper. Roll up jelly-roll style. To serve, cut into six pieces.

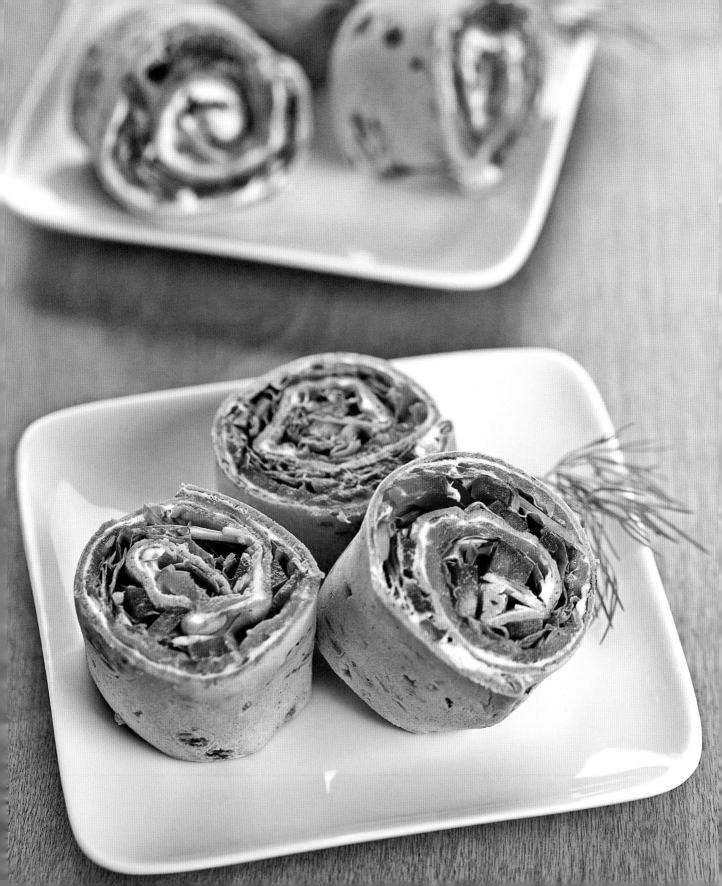

Chorizo and Caramelized Onion Tortilla

Makes 18 servings

2 tablespoons olive oil

3 medium yellow onions, sliced

½ pound Spanish chorizo (about 2 links) or andouille sausage, diced

6 eggs

Salt and black pepper

½ cup chopped fresh parsley

1. Heat oil in medium skillet over medium heat. Add onions; cook, covered, 10 minutes or until onions are translucent. Reduce heat to low; cook, uncovered, 40 minutes or until golden and very tender. Remove onions from skillet; let cool.

2. Cook chorizo in same skillet over medium heat 5 minutes or just until chorizo begins to brown, stirring occasionally. Remove chorizo from skillet; set aside to cool.

3. Preheat oven to 350°F. Spray 9-inch square baking pan with olive oil cooking spray.

4. Whisk eggs in medium bowl; season with salt and pepper. Add onions, chorizo and parsley; stir gently until well blended. Pour egg mixture into prepared pan.

5. Bake 12 to 15 minutes or until center is almost set. *Turn oven to broil.* Broil 1 to 2 minutes or until top just starts to brown. Transfer pan to wire rack; cool completely. Cut into 36 triangles or squares; serve cold or at room temperature.

Tip: The tortilla can be made up to 1 day ahead and refrigerated until serving. To serve at room temperature, remove from refrigerator 30 minutes before serving.

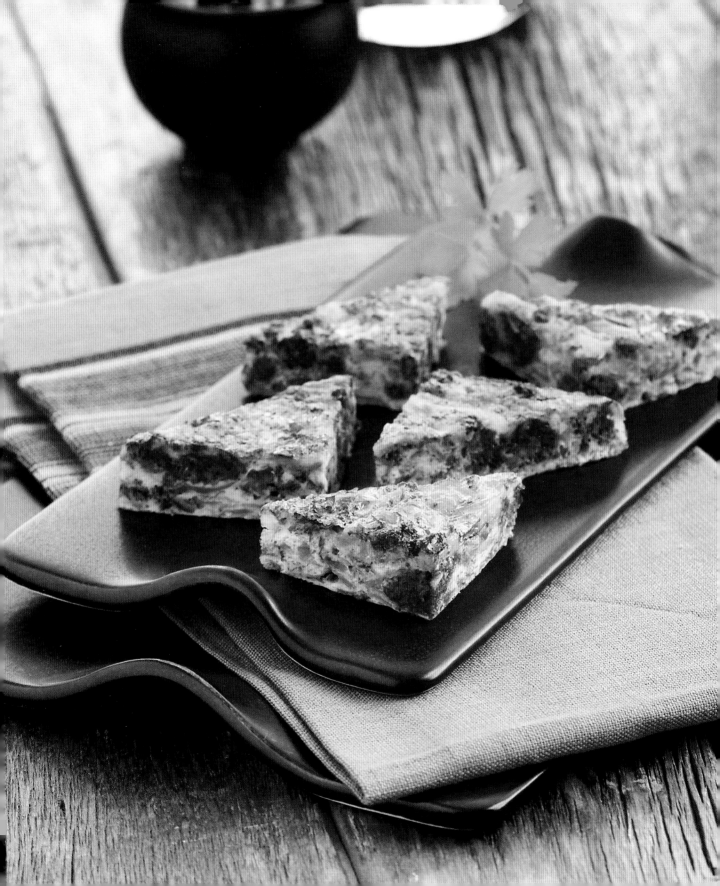

Mini Spinach Frittatas

Makes 12 mini frittatas (4 servings)

1 tablespoon olive oil

½ cup chopped onion

8 eggs

¼ cup plain yogurt

1 package (10 ounces) frozen chopped spinach, thawed and squeezed dry

½ cup (2 ounces) shredded white Cheddar cheese

¼ cup grated Parmesan cheese

¾ teaspoon salt

⅛ teaspoon black pepper

⅛ teaspoon ground red pepper

Dash ground nutmeg

1. Preheat oven to 350°F. Spray 12 standard (2½-inch) muffin cups with nonstick cooking spray.

2. Heat oil in large nonstick skillet over medium heat. Add onion; cook and stir about 5 minutes or until tender. Set aside to cool slightly.

3. Whisk eggs and yogurt in large bowl. Stir in spinach, Cheddar, Parmesan, salt, black pepper, red pepper, nutmeg and onion until blended. Divide mixture evenly among prepared muffin cups.

4. Bake 20 to 25 minutes or until eggs are puffed and firm and no longer shiny. Cool in pan 2 minutes. Loosen bottom and sides with small spatula or knife; remove to wire rack. Serve warm, cold or at room temperature.

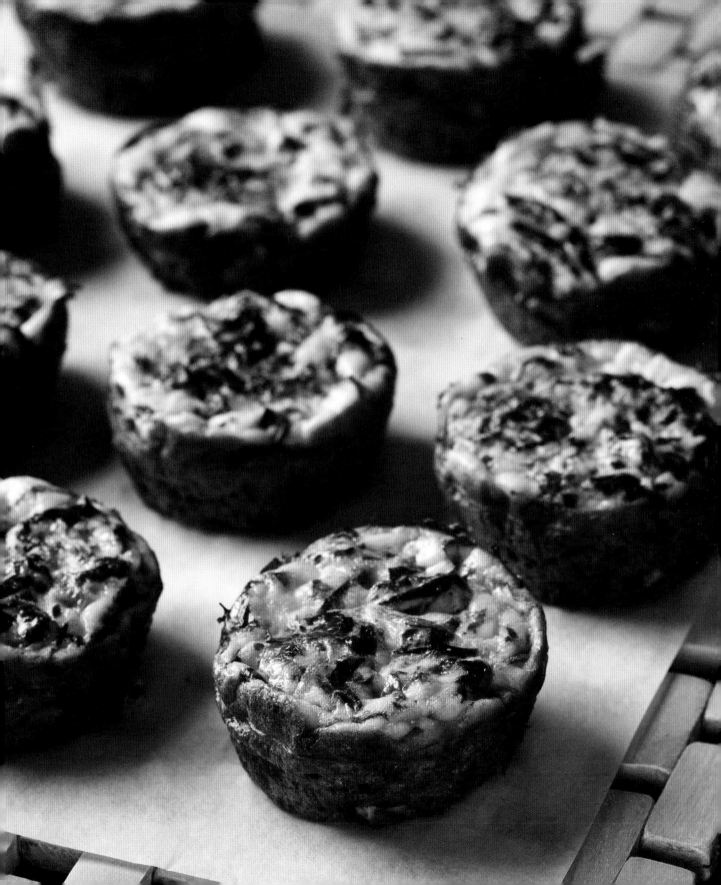

Roasted Garlic Spread with Three Cheeses

Makes about 20 servings

PER SERVING

90 calories
8g total fat
3g carbs
3g net carbs
0g dietary fiber
3g protein

2 medium heads garlic

2 packages (8 ounces each) cream cheese, softened

1 package (3½ ounces) goat cheese

2 tablespoons (1 ounce) crumbled blue cheese, plus additional for garnish

1 teaspoon dried thyme

Fresh thyme (optional)

Cut-up fresh vegetables (optional)

1. Preheat oven to 400°F. Trim top off garlic; discard. Moisten heads of garlic with water; wrap in foil. Bake 45 minutes or until garlic is softened; cool completely. Squeeze garlic into small bowl; discard skins. Mash garlic with fork.

2. Beat cream cheese and goat cheese in medium bowl until smooth. Stir in garlic, 2 tablespoons blue cheese and dried thyme. Cover and refrigerate 3 hours or overnight.

3. Spoon dip into serving bowl. Garnish with additional blue cheese and fresh thyme. Serve with fresh vegetables, if desired.

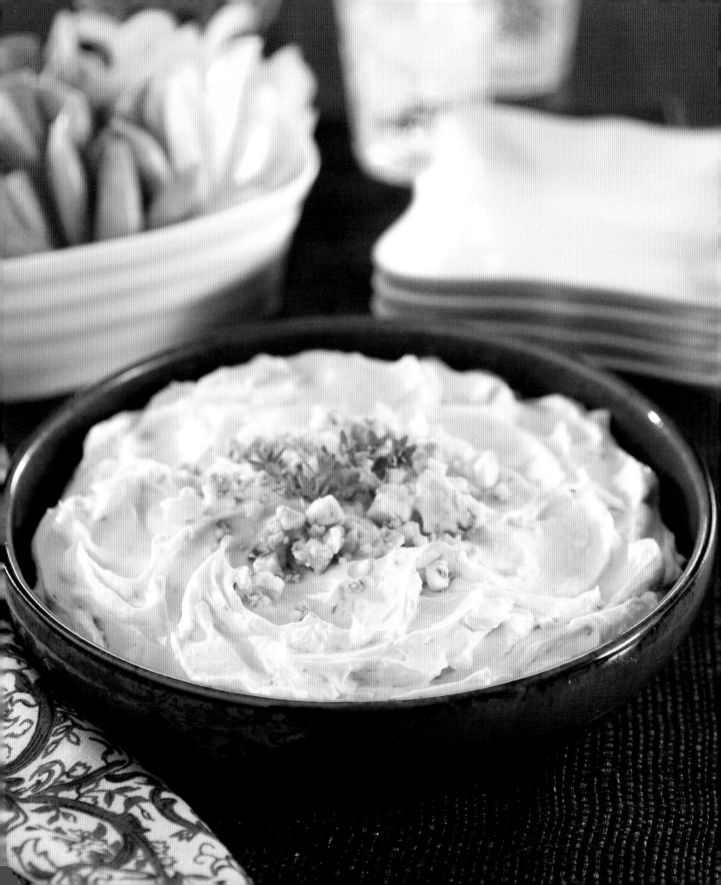

Bacon & Onion Cheese Ball

Makes 20 servings (2 tablespoons per serving)

1 package (8 ounces) cream cheese, softened

½ cup sour cream

½ cup bottled real bacon bits

½ cup chopped green onions, plus additional for garnish

¼ cup crumbled blue cheese

Celery sticks and whole wheat crackers (optional)

1. Beat cream cheese, sour cream, bacon bits, green onions and blue cheese in large bowl until well blended. Shape mixture into a ball. Wrap in plastic wrap; refrigerate at least 1 hour.

2. Place cheese ball on serving plate. Garnish with additional green onions. Serve with celery and crackers, if desired.

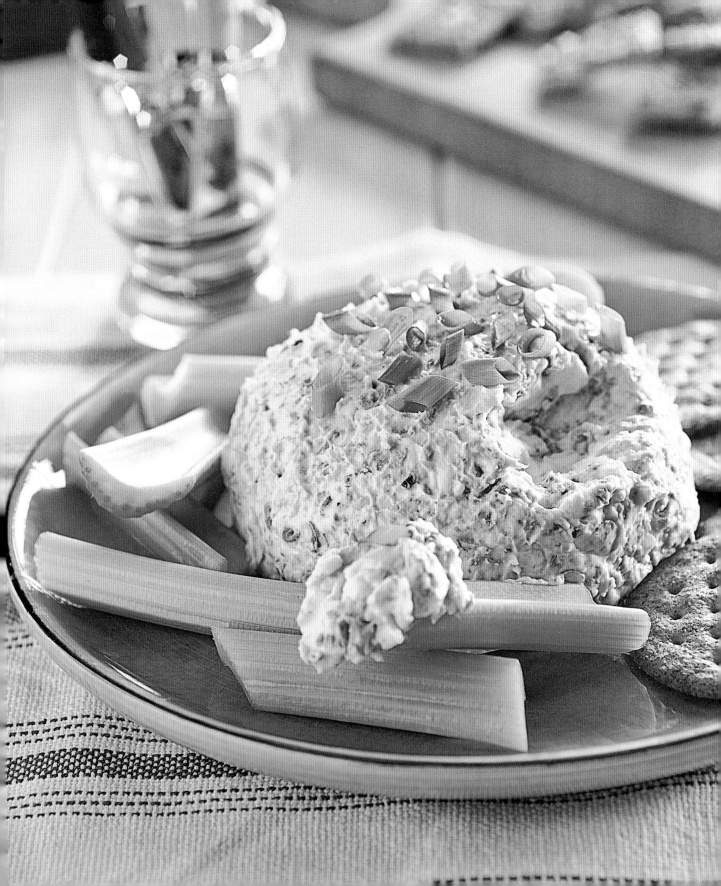

Classic Deviled Eggs

Makes 12 deviled eggs

PER SERVING

30 calories
3g **total fat**
0g **carbs**
0g **net carbs**
0g **dietary fiber**
2g **protein**

6 eggs

3 tablespoons mayonnaise

½ teaspoon apple cider vinegar

½ teaspoon yellow mustard

⅛ teaspoon salt

Optional toppings: black pepper, paprika, minced chives and/or minced red onion (optional)

1. Bring medium saucepan of water to a boil. Gently add eggs with slotted spoon. Reduce heat to maintain a simmer; cook 12 minutes. Meanwhile, fill medium bowl with cold water and ice cubes. Drain eggs and place in ice water; cool 10 minutes.

2. Carefully peel eggs. Cut eggs in half; place yolks in small bowl. Add mayonnaise, vinegar, mustard and salt; mash until well blended. Spoon mixture into egg whites; garnish with desired toppings.

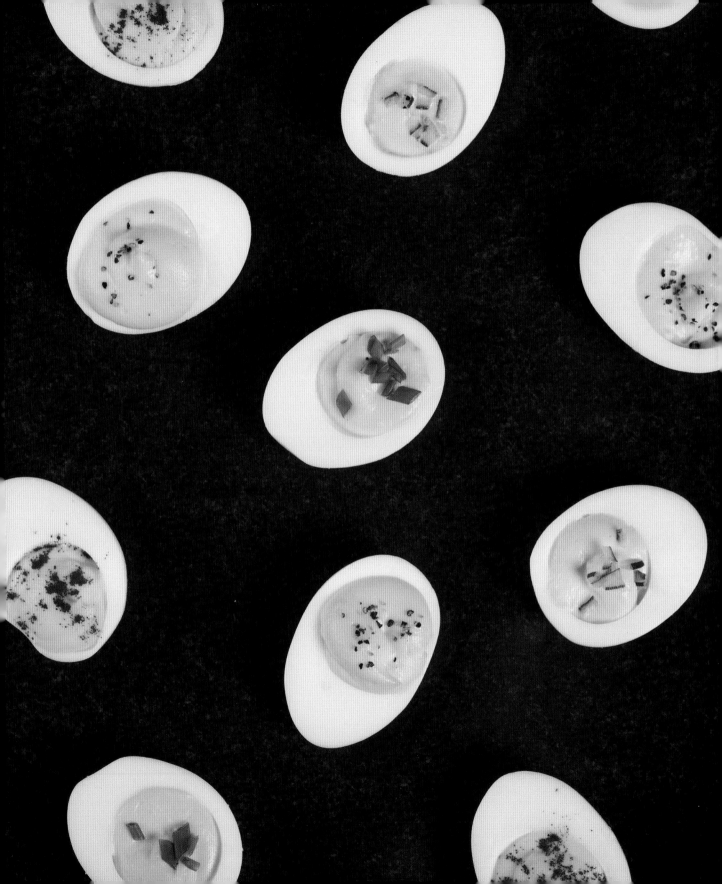

Jalapeño Poppers

Makes 20 to 24 poppers

10 to 12 fresh jalapeño peppers*

1 package (8 ounces) cream cheese, softened

1½ cups (6 ounces) shredded Cheddar cheese, divided

2 green onions, finely chopped

½ teaspoon onion powder

¼ teaspoon salt

⅛ teaspoon garlic powder

6 slices bacon, crisp-cooked and finely chopped

2 tablespoons almond flour (optional)

2 tablespoons grated Parmesan or Romano cheese

For large jalapeño peppers, use 10. For small peppers, use 12.

1. Preheat oven to 375°F. Line baking sheet with parchment paper or foil.

2. Cut each jalapeño pepper in half lengthwise; remove ribs and seeds.

3. Combine cream cheese, 1 cup Cheddar cheese, green onions, onion powder, salt and garlic powder in medium bowl. Stir in bacon. Fill each pepper half with about 1 tablespoon cheese mixture. Place on prepared baking sheet. Sprinkle with remaining ½ cup Cheddar cheese, almond flour, if desired, and Parmesan cheese.

4. Bake 10 to 12 minutes or until cheese is melted but jalapeños are still firm.

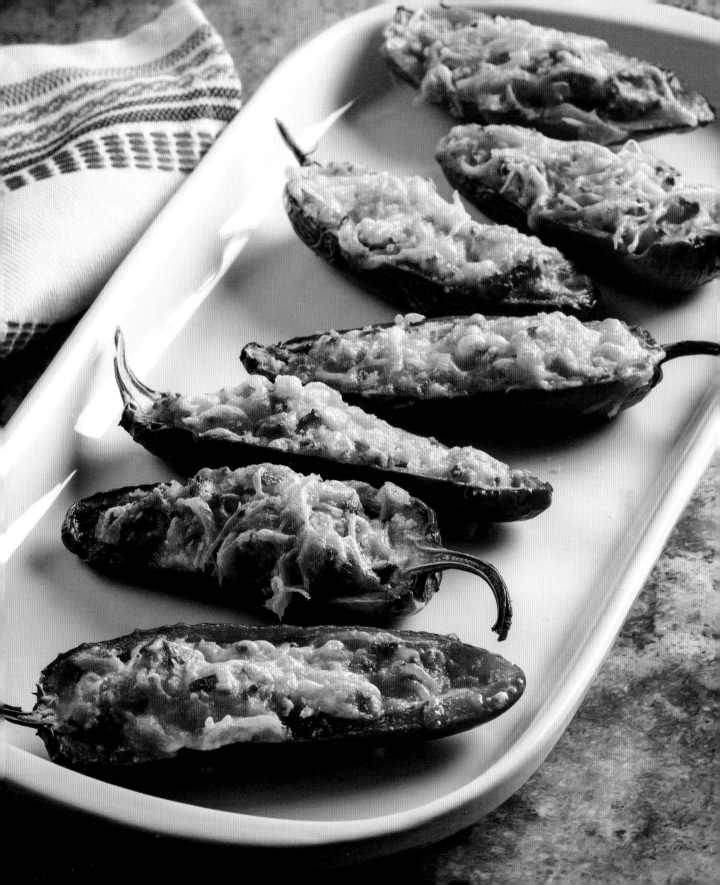

Crab Stuffed Mushrooms

Makes 12 servings

1 **pound white mushrooms (about 24 mushrooms), stems removed**

2 **cans (6 ounces each) lump crabmeat, drained**

½ **cup (2 ounces) shredded Monterey Jack cheese**

⅓ **cup finely chopped green onions**

3 **tablespoons mayonnaise**

2 **tablespoons shredded Parmesan cheese**

1 **tablespoon Worcestershire sauce**

1 **teaspoon minced garlic**

2 **tablespoons almond flour**

1. Preheat oven to 350°F. Line baking sheet with parchment paper. Place mushrooms, tops sides down, on prepared baking sheet.

2. Combine crabmeat, Monterey Jack cheese, green onions, mayonnaise, Parmesan cheese, Worcestershire sauce and garlic in medium bowl; gently mix. Spoon evenly into mushroom caps, flattening slightly, if necessary. Top evenly with almond flour.

3. Bake 20 minutes or until lightly browned.

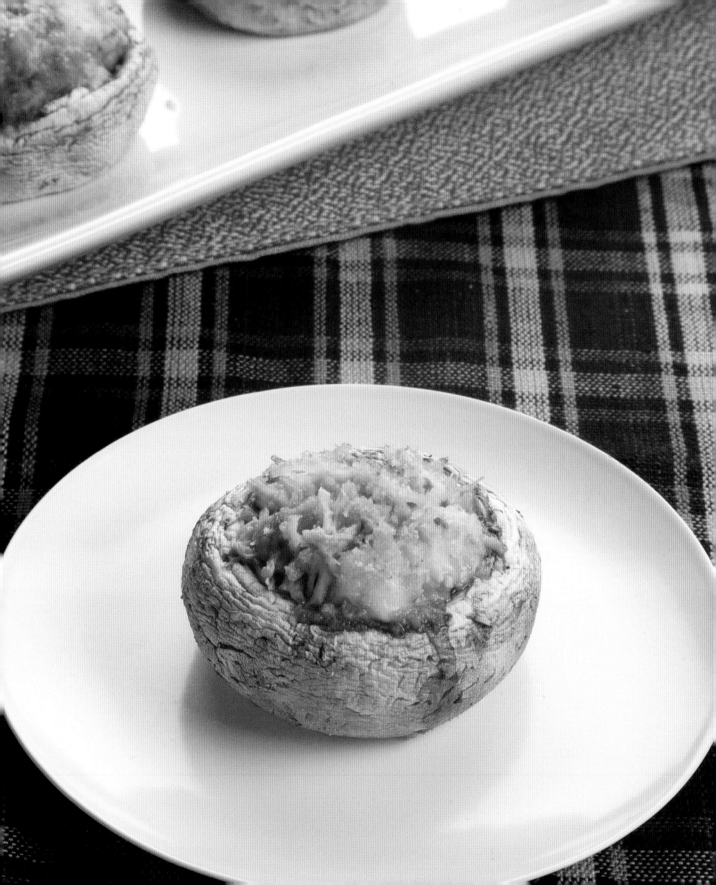

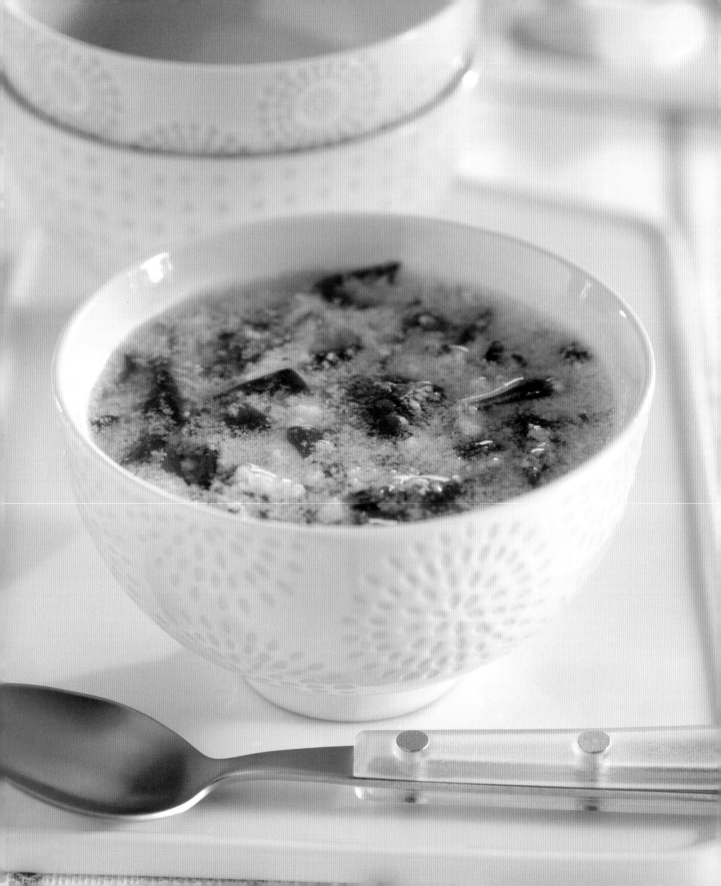

soups & chilis

PER SERVING

46 calories
1g **total fat**
4g **carbs**
3g **net carbs**
1g **dietary fiber**
6g **protein**

Roman Spinach Soup

Makes 8 servings

6 cups chicken broth

1 cup cholesterol-free egg substitute

¼ cup minced fresh basil

3 tablespoons grated Parmesan cheese

2 tablespoons fresh lemon juice

1 tablespoon minced fresh parsley

¼ teaspoon white pepper

⅛ teaspoon ground nutmeg

8 cups packed fresh spinach, chopped

1. Bring broth to a boil in 4-quart saucepan over medium heat.

2. Beat together egg substitute, basil, Parmesan cheese, lemon juice, parsley, white pepper and nutmeg in small bowl. Set aside.

3. Stir spinach into broth; simmer 1 minute. Slowly pour egg mixture into broth mixture, whisking constantly so egg threads form. Simmer 2 to 3 minutes or until egg is cooked. Serve immediately.

Note: Soup may look curdled.

Chilled Cucumber Soup

Makes 4 servings

1 large cucumber, peeled, seeded and coarsely chopped

¾ cup plain nonfat Greek yogurt

¼ cup packed fresh dill

½ teaspoon salt (optional)

⅛ teaspoon ground white pepper (optional)

1½ cups chicken or vegetable broth

4 fresh dill sprigs

1. Place cucumber in blender or food processor; process until finely chopped. Add yogurt, ¼ cup dill, salt and pepper, if desired; process until smooth.

2. Transfer mixture to large bowl; stir in broth. Cover and refrigerate at least 2 hours or up to 24 hours. Ladle into bowls; garnish with dill sprigs.

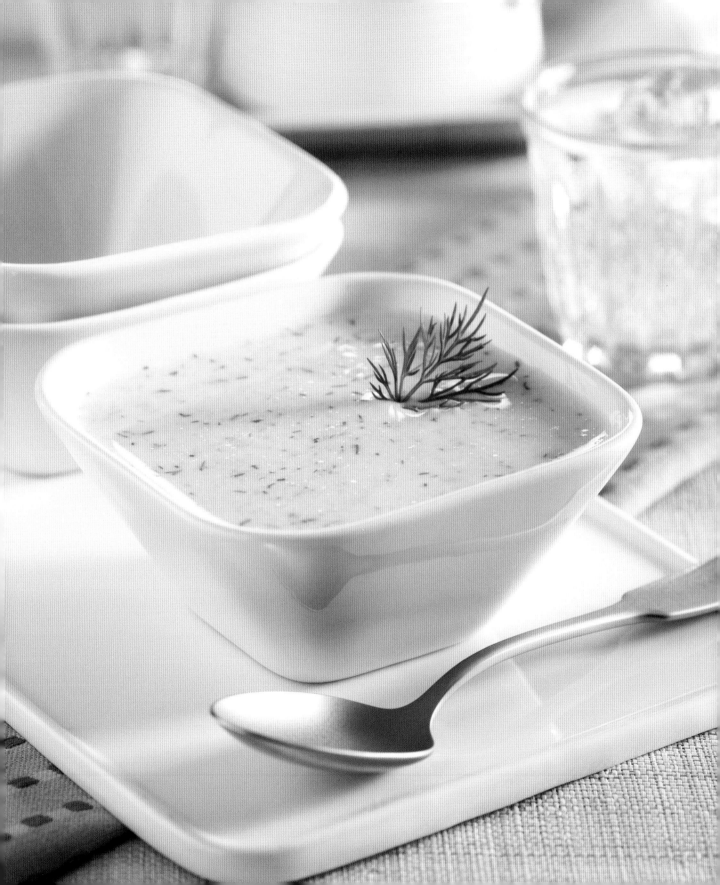

Chilled Fresh Tomato Basil Soup

Makes 4 servings

- 3 medium tomatoes, diced
- 1 cup finely chopped green bell pepper
- ½ medium cucumber, peeled, seeded and finely chopped
- ¼ cup chopped fresh basil
- ¼ cup finely chopped peperoncinis
- 1 cup water
- 3 tablespoons red wine vinegar
- ½ teaspoon salt
- 2 tablespoons chopped fresh parsley
- 2 tablespoons extra virgin olive oil

Combine tomatoes, bell pepper, cucumber, basil, peperoncinis, water, vinegar, salt, parsley and oil in medium bowl; stir to blend. Cover; refrigerate 30 minutes.

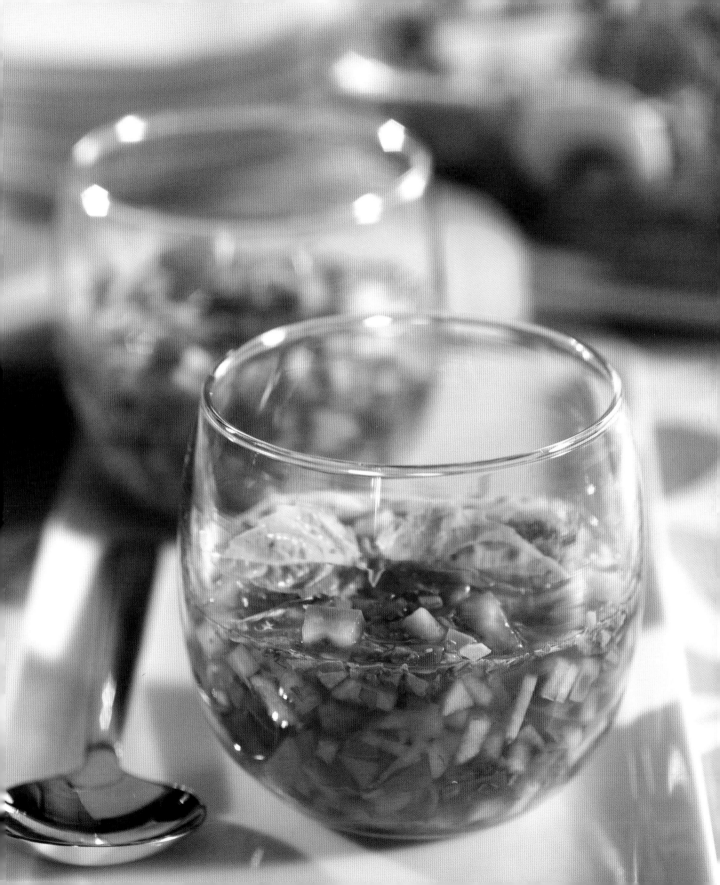

Chipotle Seafood Chili

Makes 4 servings

PER SERVING

192 calories
6g **total fat**
10g **carbs**
8g **net carbs**
2g **dietary fiber**
24g **protein**

1 **tablespoon canola or vegetable oil**

1 **small green bell pepper, chopped**

½ **cup chopped onion**

4 **cloves garlic, minced**

1 **can (about 14 ounces) fire-roasted diced tomatoes, undrained**

½ **cup chicken or vegetable broth**

1 **tablespoon canned chipotle peppers in adobo sauce,* puréed**

1 **teaspoon ground coriander**

8 **ounces fresh bay scallops**

6 **ounces raw medium shrimp**

Lime wedges (optional)

Fresh cilantro (optional)

These (7-ounce cans) can be found in the Mexican section of the grocery store near the refried beans and salsas. Purée the entire can of chipotle peppers in a blender. Refrigerate or freeze remaining puréed peppers for another use.

1. Heat oil in large saucepan over medium heat. Add bell pepper and onion; cook and stir 5 minutes. Add garlic; cook and stir 30 seconds.

2. Add tomatoes with their juices, broth and chipotle peppers; bring just to a boil over medium heat. Reduce heat; simmer uncovered 5 minutes or until vegetables are tender.

3. Sprinkle coriander over scallops and shrimp; stir into tomato mixture. Simmer 5 minutes or until seafood is opaque and just cooked through. Ladle into shallow bowls; garnish with lime and cilantro, if desired.

Note: Cilantro is a versatile herb often used in soups and chilis. Its distinctive flavor complements spicy foods, especially Mexican, Caribbean, Thai, and Vietnamese dishes.

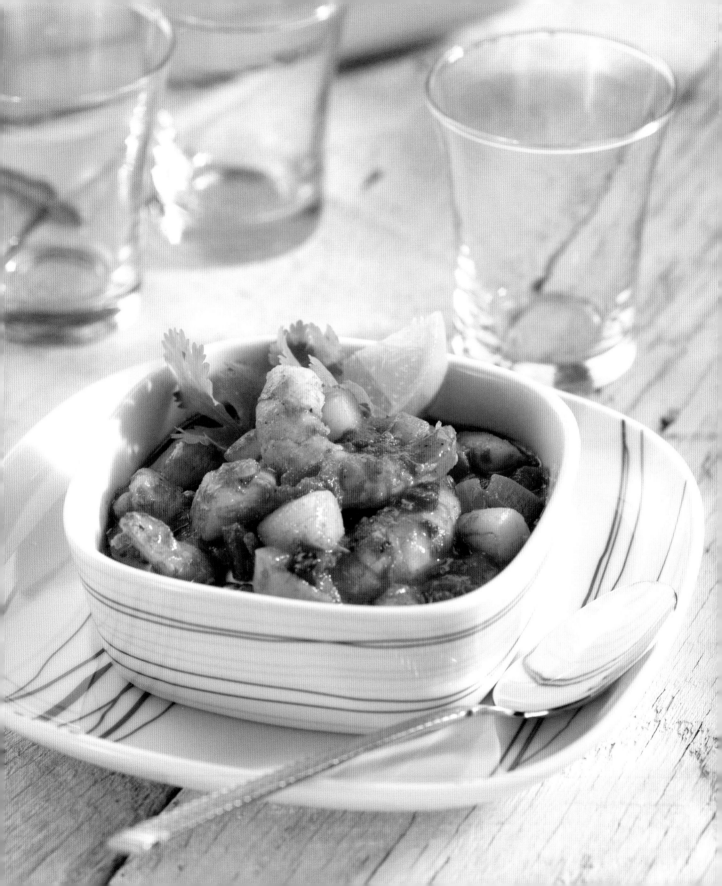

Chicken Tortilla Soup

Makes 8 servings

- 1 whole chicken (about 3½ pounds), giblets removed
- 5 cups chicken broth
- 1 cup chopped onion
- 1 clove garlic, minced
- 1 teaspoon ground cumin
- 1 can (about 14 ounces) diced tomatoes
- 1 can (4 ounces) diced mild or hot green chiles
- ⅓ cup chopped fresh cilantro
- Juice of 1 lime
- 1 avocado, diced
- ½ cup tortilla strips (optional)

Slow Cooker Directions

1. Place whole chicken, broth, onion, garlic and cumin in slow cooker. Cover; cook on HIGH 4½ to 5 hours or until chicken is tender and falling off of bones. Remove chicken from slow cooker; set aside to cool slightly. Meanwhile, skim fat from top of broth and discard.

2. When chicken is cool enough to handle, shred using two forks. Discard any excess fat and bone. Return shredded chicken to slow cooker. Add tomatoes, green chiles, cilantro and lime juice.

3. Cover; cook on HIGH 30 to 60 minutes. Ladle soup into bowls; top with avocado and tortilla strips, if desired.

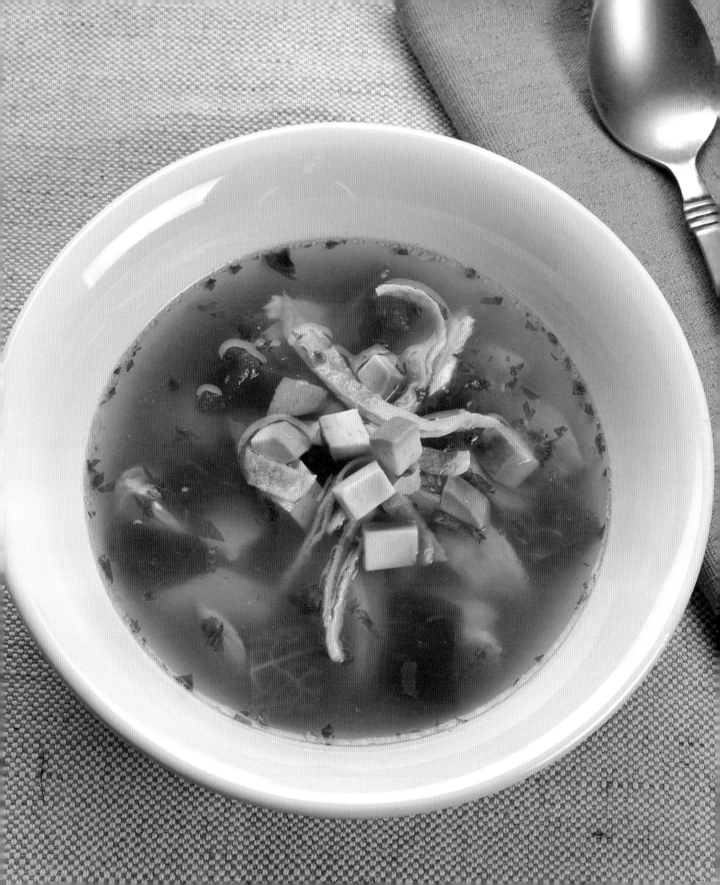

Stir-Fry Beef & Vegetable Soup

Makes 6 servings

1 boneless beef top sirloin or top round steak (about 1 pound)

2 teaspoons dark sesame oil, divided

3 cans (about 14 ounces each) beef broth

1 package (16 ounces) frozen stir-fry vegetables

3 green onions, thinly sliced

¼ cup stir-fry sauce

1. Slice beef lengthwise in half, then crosswise into ⅛-inch-thick strips.

2. Heat 1 teaspoon oil in large saucepan or Dutch oven over medium-high heat; tilt pan to coat bottom. Add half of beef in single layer. Cook 1 minute, without stirring, until lightly browned on bottom. Turn and cook other side about 1 minute. Remove beef from saucepan. Repeat with remaining 1 teaspoon oil and beef; set aside.

3. Add broth to saucepan. Cover; bring to a boil over high heat. Add vegetables. Reduce heat; simmer 3 to 5 minutes or until vegetables are heated through. Add beef, green onions and stir-fry sauce; simmer 1 minute.

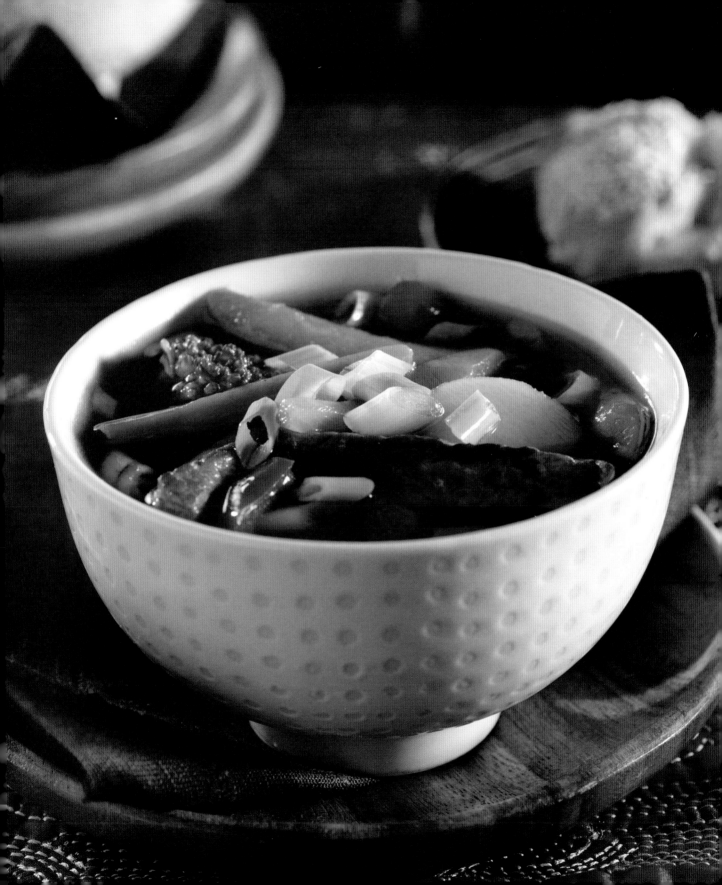

Tex-Mex Chili

Makes 6 servings

PER SERVING

290 **calories**
14g **total fat**
5g **carbs**
3g **net carbs**
2g **dietary fiber**
35g **protein**

4 slices bacon, diced

2 pounds boneless beef top round or chuck shoulder steak, trimmed and cut into ½-inch cubes

1 medium onion, chopped

2 cloves garlic, minced

¼ cup chili powder

1 teaspoon salt

1 teaspoon dried oregano

1 teaspoon ground cumin

½ to 1 teaspoon ground red pepper

½ teaspoon hot pepper sauce

4 cups water

Additional chopped onion (optional)

1. Cook bacon in Dutch oven over medium-high heat until crisp. Drain on paper towel-lined plate.

2. Add half of beef to drippings in Dutch oven; cook and stir until lightly browned. Remove beef to plate; repeat with remaining beef.

3. Add onion and garlic to Dutch oven; cook and stir over medium heat 3 minutes or until onion is tender. Return beef and bacon to Dutch oven. Stir in chili powder, salt, oregano, cumin, red pepper and hot pepper sauce; mix well. Stir in water; bring to a boil over high heat.

4. Reduce heat to low; cover and simmer 1½ hours. Skim fat from surface; simmer, uncovered, 30 minutes or until beef is very tender and chili has thickened slightly. Garnish with additional chopped onion.

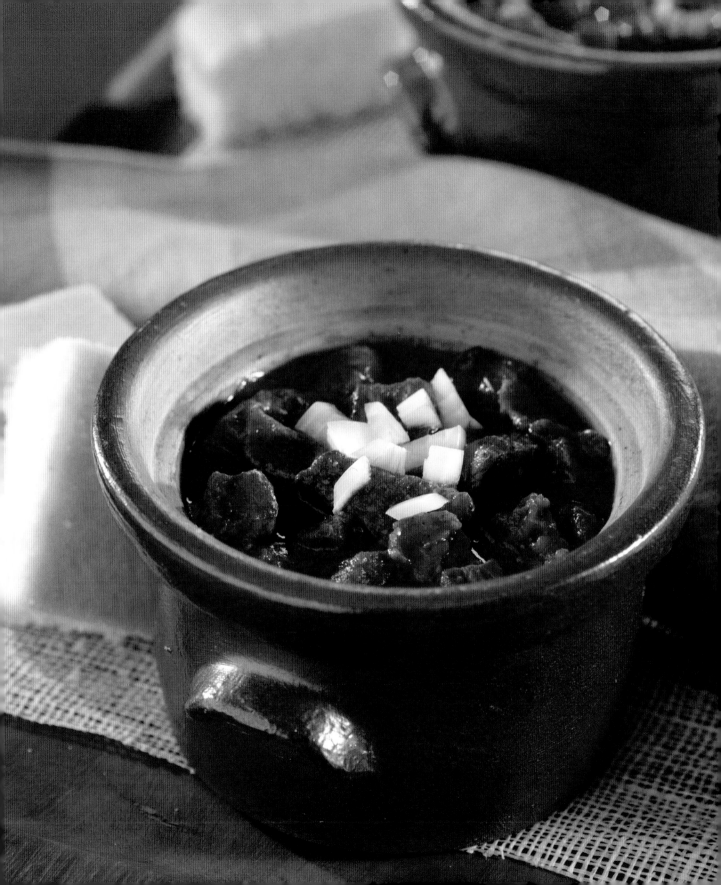

Egg Drop Soup

Makes 2 servings

PER SERVING

45 calories
1g **total fat**
3g **carbs**
2g **net carbs**
1g **dietary fiber**
7g **protein**

2 cans (about 14 ounces each) chicken broth

1 tablespoon soy sauce

2 teaspoons cornstarch

½ cup cholesterol-free egg substitute

¼ cup thinly sliced green onions

1. Bring broth to a boil in large saucepan over high heat. Reduce heat to medium-low.

2. Whisk soy sauce and cornstarch in small bowl until smooth and well blended; stir into broth. Cook and stir 2 minutes or until slightly thickened.

3. Stirring constantly in one direction, slowly pour egg substitute in thin stream into soup.

4. Ladle soup into bowls; sprinkle with green onions.

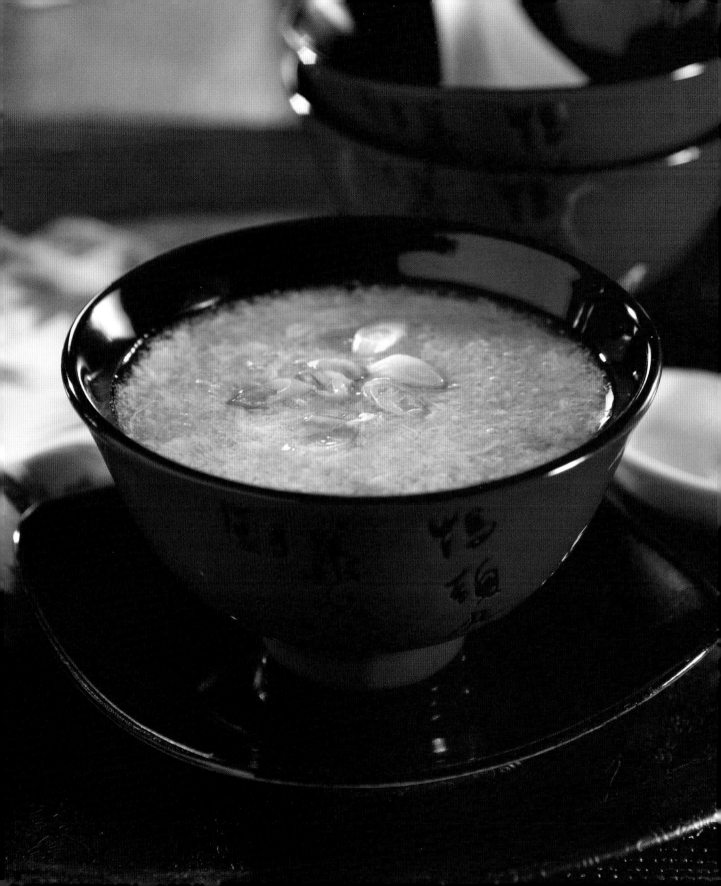

Cheesy Broccoli Soup

Makes 2 servings

PER SERVING

400 calories
34g **total fat**
12g **carbs**
9g **net carbs**
3g **dietary fiber**
11g **protein**

½ teaspoon olive oil

¼ cup finely chopped onion

1 cup chicken broth

3 cups small broccoli florets or thawed frozen chopped broccoli

½ cup whipping cream

⅛ teaspoon ground red pepper

2 ounces cubed pasteurized process cheese product

¼ cup sour cream

⅛ teaspoon salt

1. Heat oil in medium saucepan over medium-high heat. Add onion; cook and stir 4 minutes or until translucent.

2. Add broth; bring to a boil over high heat. Add broccoli; return to a boil. Reduce heat to low; cover and simmer 5 minutes or until broccoli is tender.

3. Whisk in cream and red pepper. Remove from heat; stir in cheese product until melted. Stir in sour cream and salt.

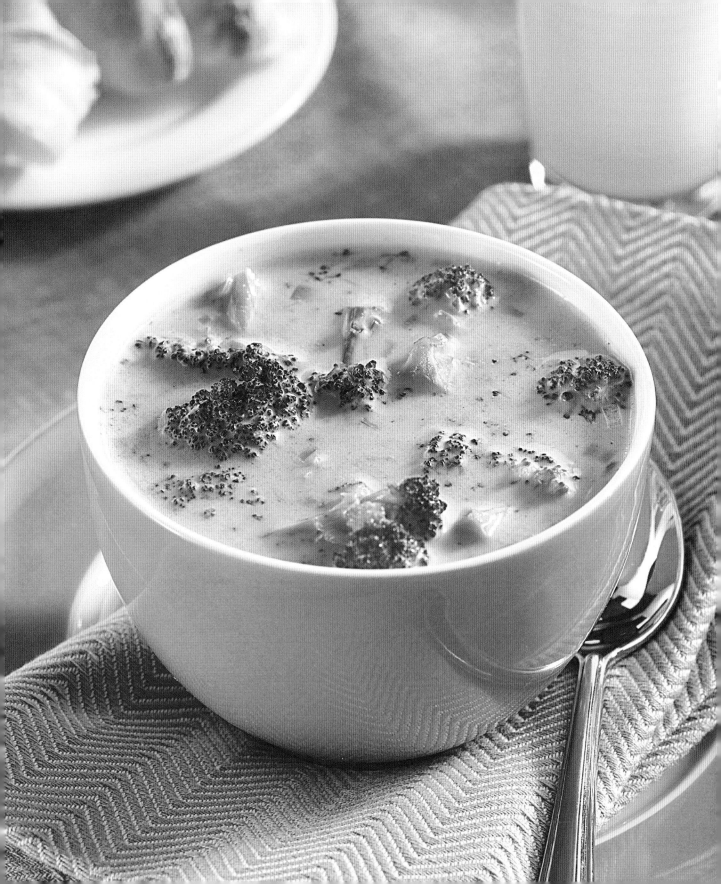

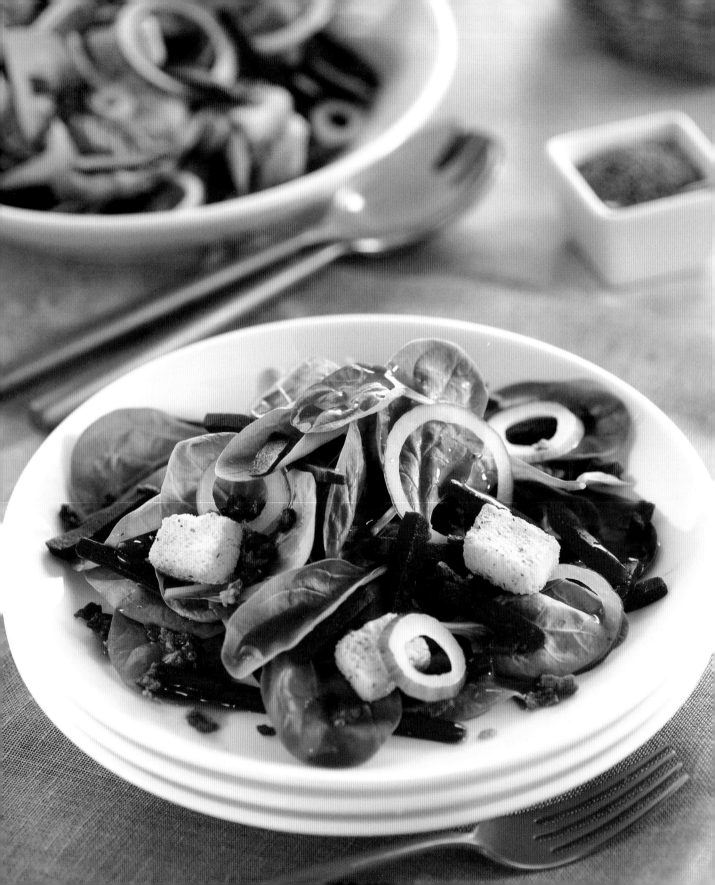

salads

PER SERVING

80 calories
3g **total fat**
9g **carbs**
7g **net carbs**
2g **dietary fiber**
5g **protein**

Spinach Salad with Beets

Makes 4 servings

6 cups (6 ounces) packed baby spinach or torn spinach leaves

1 cup canned pickled julienned beets, drained

¼ cup thinly sliced red onion, separated into rings

¼ cup fat-free croutons

⅓ cup low-fat raspberry vinaigrette salad dressing

¼ cup real bacon bits

Black pepper (optional)

1. Combine spinach, beets, onion and croutons in large bowl. Add dressing; toss to coat.

2. Divide evenly among four serving plates. Sprinkle with bacon bits and pepper, if desired.

Thai Grilled Beef Salad

Makes 4 servings

PER SERVING

200 **calories**
6g **total fat**
7g **carbs**
4g **net carbs**
3g **dietary fiber**
26g **protein**

3 tablespoons Thai seasoning blend, divided

1 beef flank steak (about 1 pound)

2 tablespoons chopped fresh cilantro

2 tablespoons chopped fresh basil

2 red Thai chile peppers *or* 1 red jalapeño pepper,* seeded and sliced into thin slivers

1 tablespoon finely chopped lemongrass

1 tablespoon minced red onion

1 clove garlic, minced

Juice of 1 lime

1 tablespoon fish sauce

1 large carrot, grated

1 cucumber, chopped

4 cups assorted salad greens

*Thai chile peppers and jalapeño peppers can sting and irritate the skin, so wear rubber gloves when handling peppers and do not touch your eyes.

1. Prepare grill for direct cooking.

2. Sprinkle 1 tablespoon Thai seasoning over beef; turn to coat. Cover and marinate 15 minutes. Place steak on grid over medium heat. Grill, uncovered, 17 to 21 minutes for medium rare to medium or until desired doneness, turning once. Cool 10 minutes.

3. Meanwhile, combine remaining 2 tablespoons Thai seasoning, cilantro, basil, chile peppers, lemongrass, onion, garlic, lime juice and fish sauce in medium bowl; mix well.

4. Thinly slice beef across grain. Add beef, carrot and cucumber to dressing; toss to coat. Arrange on bed of greens.

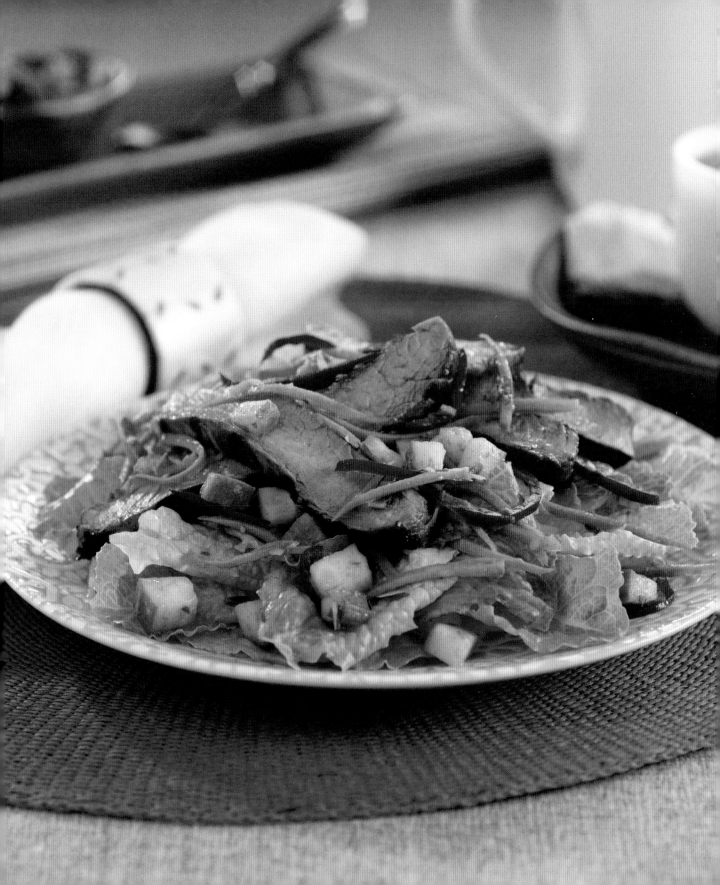

Cobb Salad to Go

Makes 4 servings

- ½ cup blue cheese salad dressing
- 1 ripe avocado, diced
- 1 tomato, chopped
- 6 ounces cooked chicken breast, cut into 1-inch pieces
- 4 slices bacon, crisp-cooked and crumbled
- 2 hard-cooked eggs, mashed
- 1 large carrot, shredded
- ½ cup blue cheese, crumbled
- 1 package (10 ounces) torn mixed salad greens

1. Place 2 tablespoons salad dressing into bottom of four (1-quart) jars. Layer remaining ingredients on top, ending with salad greens. Seal jars.

2. Refrigerate until ready to serve.

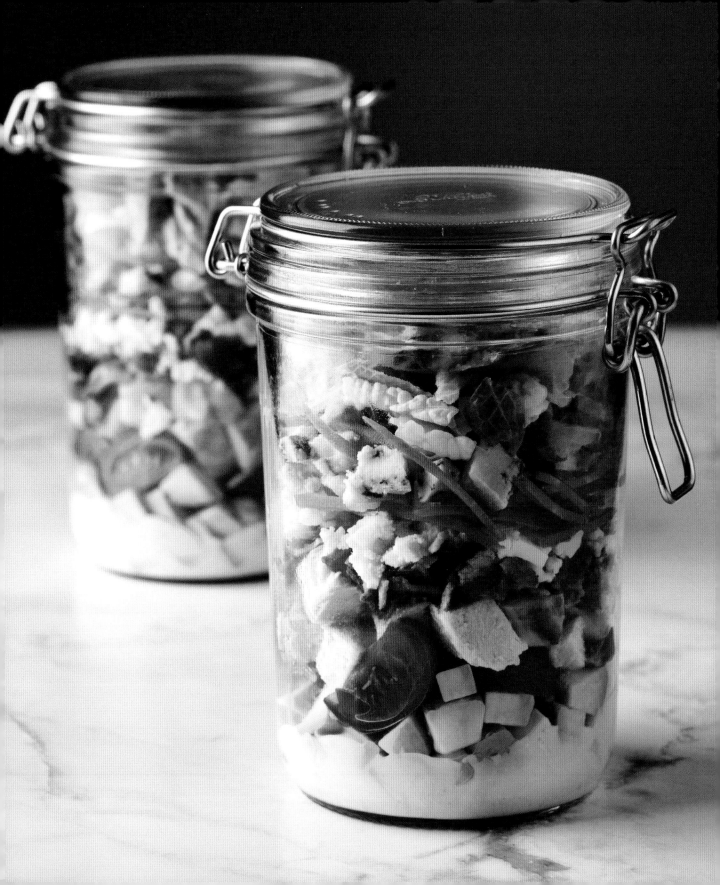

Green Goddess Cobb Salad

Makes 6 servings

PER SERVING

750 **calories**
62g **total fat**
14g **carbs**
8g **net carbs**
6g **dietary fiber**
40g **protein**

Pickled Onions

- 1 cup thinly sliced red onion
- ½ cup white wine vinegar
- ¼ cup water
- 1 teaspoon salt

Dressing

- 1 cup mayonnaise
- 1 cup fresh Italian parsley leaves
- 1 cup baby arugula
- ¼ cup extra virgin olive oil
- 3 tablespoons lemon juice
- 3 tablespoons minced fresh chives
- 2 tablespoons fresh tarragon leaves
- 1 clove garlic, minced
- 1 teaspoon Dijon mustard
- ½ teaspoon salt
- ⅛ teaspoon black pepper

Salad

- 4 eggs
- 4 cups Italian salad blend (romaine and radicchio)
- 2 cups chopped stemmed kale
- 2 cups baby arugula
- 2 avocados, halved and sliced
- 2 tomatoes, cut into wedges
- 2 cups cooked chicken strips
- 1 cup chopped crisp-cooked bacon

1. For pickled onions, combine onion, vinegar, ¼ cup water and 1 teaspoon salt in large glass jar. Seal jar; shake well. Refrigerate at least 1 hour or up to 1 week.

2. For dressing, combine mayonnaise, parsley, 1 cup arugula, oil, lemon juice, chives, tarragon, garlic, mustard, ½ teaspoon salt and pepper in blender or food processor; blend until smooth, stopping to scrape down side once or twice. Transfer to jar; refrigerate until ready to use. Just before serving, thin dressing with 1 to 2 tablespoons water, if necessary, to reach desired consistency.

3. Fill medium saucepan with water; bring to a boil over high heat. Carefully lower eggs into water. Reduce heat to medium; boil gently 12 minutes. Drain eggs; add cold water and ice cubes to saucepan to cool eggs. When eggs are cool enough to handle, peel and cut in half lengthwise.

4. For salad, combine salad blend, kale, 2 cups arugula and pickled onions in large bowl; divide among six serving bowls. Top each salad with avocados, tomatoes, chicken, bacon and eggs. Top with ¼ cup dressing; toss to coat.

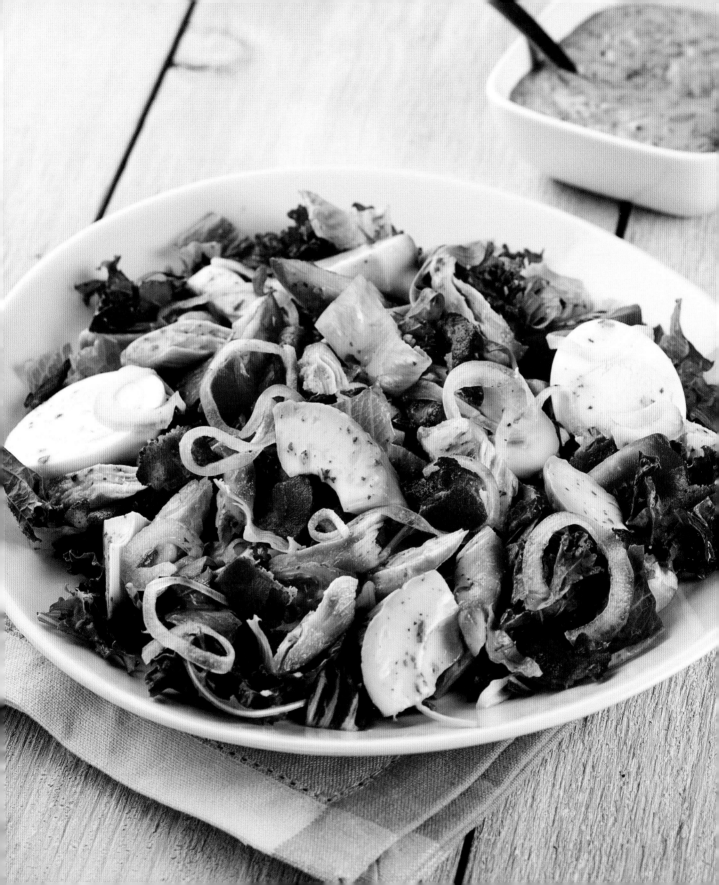

Wedge Salad

Makes 4 servings

Dressing

- ¾ cup mayonnaise
- ½ cup buttermilk
- 1 cup crumbled blue cheese, divided
- 1 clove garlic, minced
- ⅛ teaspoon onion powder
- ⅛ teaspoon salt
- ⅛ teaspoon ground black pepper

Salad

- 1 head iceberg lettuce
- 1 large tomato, diced (about 1 cup)
- ½ small red onion, cut into thin rings
- ½ cup crumbled crisp-cooked bacon (6 slices)

1. For dressing, combine mayonnaise, buttermilk, ½ cup cheese, garlic, onion powder, salt and pepper in food processor or blender; process until smooth.

2. For salad, cut lettuce into quarters through stem end; remove stem from each wedge. Place wedges on four individual serving plates; top with dressing. Sprinkle with tomato, onion, remaining ½ cup cheese and bacon.

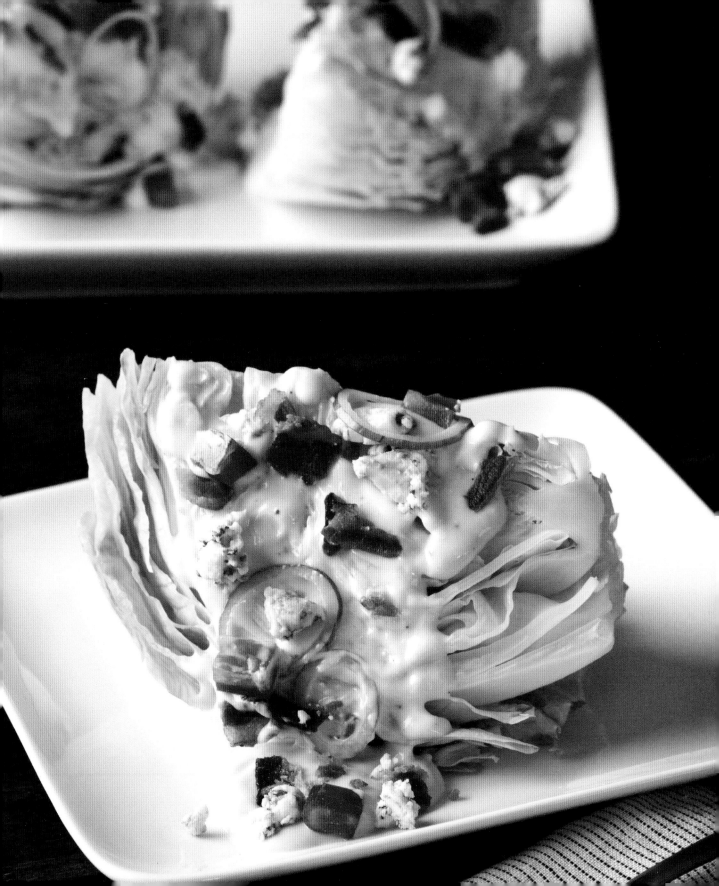

Colorful Coleslaw

Makes 8 servings

PER SERVING

100 **calories**
7g **total fat**
10g **carbs**
6g **net carbs**
4g **dietary fiber**
1g **protein**

¼ **head green cabbage, shredded or thinly sliced**

¼ **head red cabbage, shredded or thinly sliced**

1 **small yellow or orange bell pepper, thinly sliced**

1 **small jicama, peeled and julienned**

¼ **cup thinly sliced green onions**

2 **tablespoons chopped fresh cilantro**

¼ **cup vegetable oil**

¼ **cup fresh lime juice**

1 **teaspoon salt**

⅛ **teaspoon black pepper**

1. Combine cabbage, bell pepper, jicama, green onions and cilantro in large bowl.

2. Whisk oil, lime juice, salt and black pepper in small bowl until well blended. Pour over vegetables; toss to coat. Cover and refrigerate 2 to 6 hours for flavors to blend.

Note: This coleslaw makes a great topping for tacos and sandwiches.

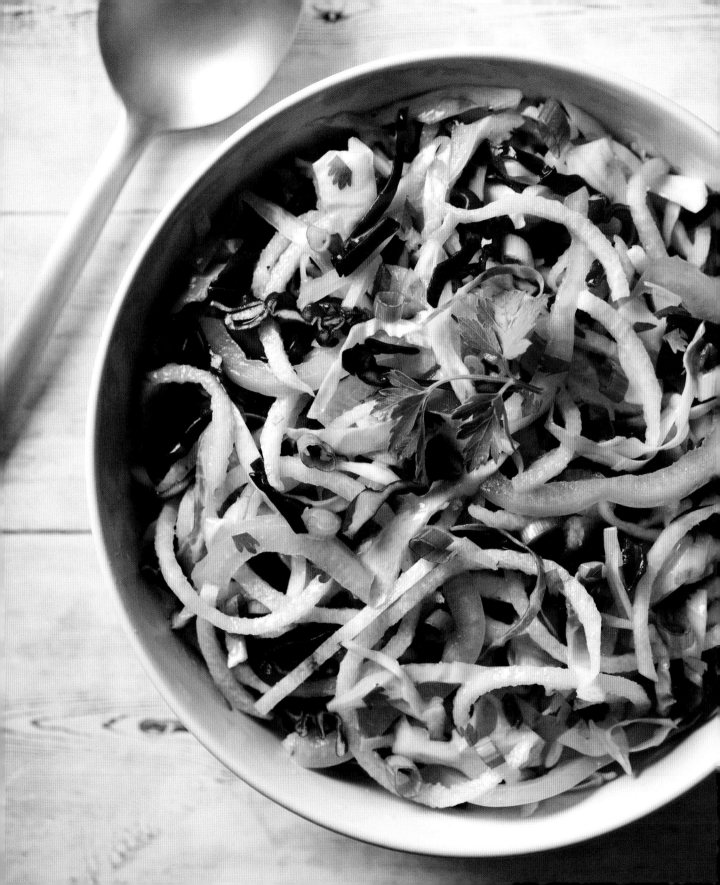

Garbage Salad

Makes 4 servings

Dressing

- ⅓ cup red wine vinegar
- 2 cloves garlic, minced
- 1 teaspoon Italian seasoning
- ¼ teaspoon salt
- ¼ teaspoon black pepper
- ⅓ cup olive oil

Salad

- 1 package (5 ounces) spring mix
- 5 romaine lettuce leaves, chopped
- 1 small cucumber, diced
- 2 small plum tomatoes, diced
- ½ red onion, thinly sliced
- ¼ cup pitted kalamata olives
- 4 radishes, thinly sliced
- 4 ounces thinly sliced Genoa salami, cut into ¼-inch strips
- 4 ounces provolone cheese, cut into ¼-inch strips
- ¼ cup grated Parmesan cheese

1. For dressing, whisk vinegar, garlic, Italian seasoning, salt and pepper in small bowl until blended. Slowly whisk in oil in thin steady stream until well blended.

2. Combine spring mix, romaine, cucumber, tomatoes, onion, olives and radishes in large bowl. Add half of dressing; toss gently to coat. Top with salami and provolone; sprinkle with Parmesan. Serve with remaining dressing.

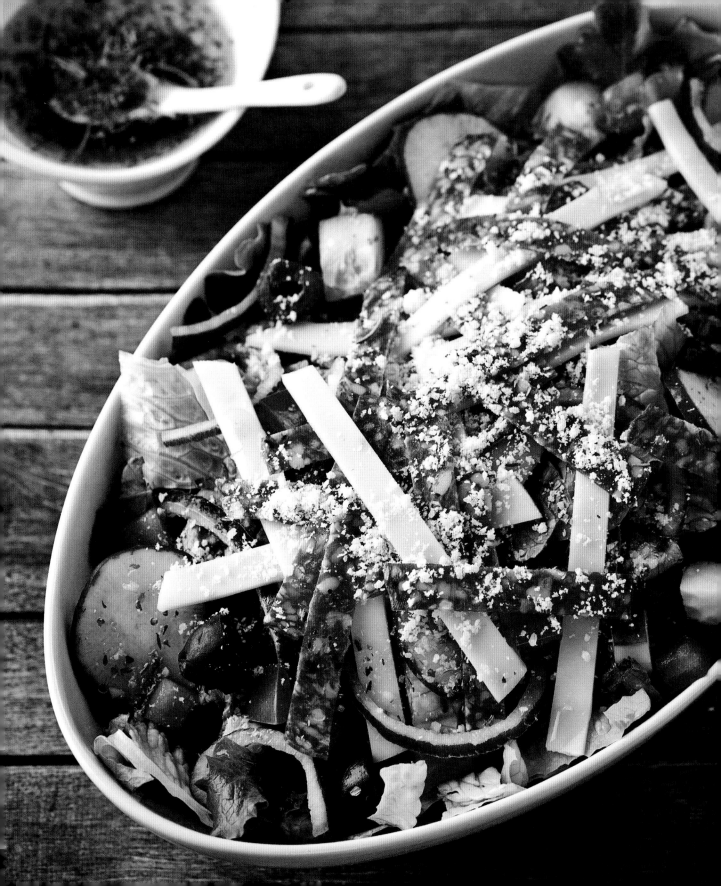

Chicken Salad Bowl

Makes 4 servings

PER SERVING

570 **calories**
44g **total fat**
18g **carbs**
9g **net carbs**
9g **dietary fiber**
30g **protein**

Chicken

- 3 tablespoons olive oil, divided
- 1 teaspoon salt
- 1 teaspoon dried oregano
- 1 teaspoon paprika
- ½ teaspoon black pepper
- 1 clove garlic, minced
- 1 pound chicken tenders, cut in half

Salad and Dressing

- ⅓ cup olive oil
- 3 tablespoons red wine vinegar
- 1 clove garlic, minced
  Salt and black pepper
- 1 cup grape tomatoes, halved
- 1 cucumber, halved crosswise and cut into sticks
- 1 red bell pepper, sliced
- 2 avocados, thinly sliced
- 2 radishes, thinly sliced
  Leaf lettuce and arugula
  Black and white sesame seeds (optional)

1. Combine 1 tablespoon oil, 1 teaspoon salt, oregano, paprika, ½ teaspoon black pepper and 1 clove garlic in large bowl. Add chicken; toss until well blended.

2. Heat remaining 2 tablespoons oil in large skillet over medium-high heat. Add chicken; cook 8 to 10 minutes or until no longer pink, turning once.

3. For dressing, whisk ⅓ cup oil, vinegar and 1 clove garlic in small bowl. Season to taste with salt and black pepper.

4. Place tomatoes, cucumber, bell pepper, avocados, radishes, lettuce and arugula in serving bowls; drizzle with dressing. Slice chicken and place on salads. Sprinkle with sesame seeds, if desired.

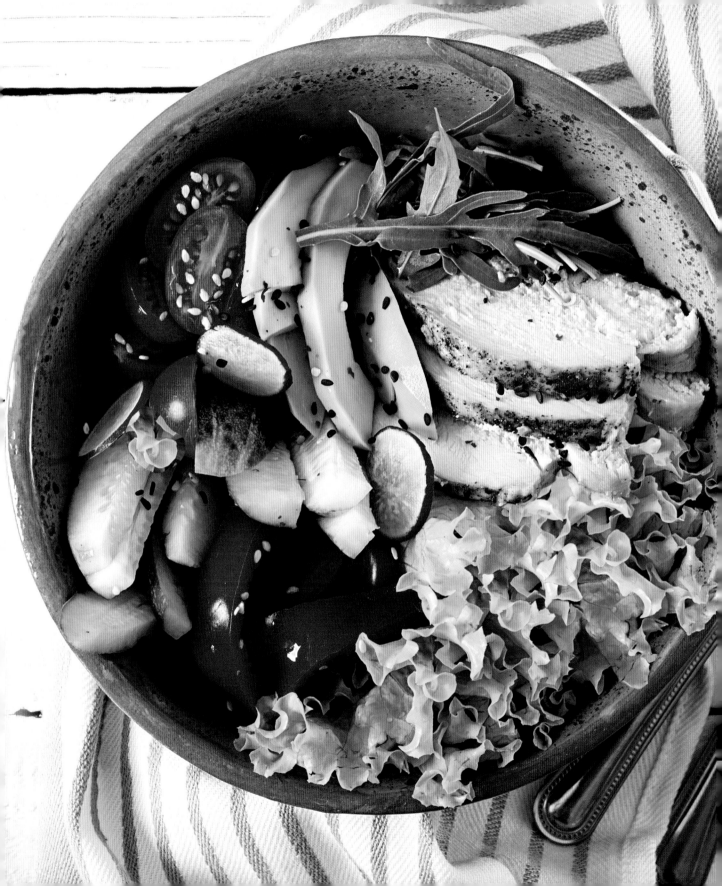

Cauliflower Picnic Salad

Makes 6 servings

2 teaspoons salt

1 head cauliflower, cut into 1-inch florets

¾ cup mayonnaise

1 tablespoon yellow mustard

2 tablespoons minced fresh parsley

⅓ cup chopped dill pickle

⅓ cup minced red onion

2 hard-cooked eggs, chopped

Salt and black pepper

1. Fill large saucepan with 1 inch water. Bring to a simmer over medium-high heat; stir in salt. Add cauliflower; reduce heat to medium. Cover and cook 5 to 7 minutes or until cauliflower is fork-tender but not mushy. Drain and cool slightly.

2. Whisk mayonnaise, mustard and parsley in large bowl. Stir in pickle and onion. Gently fold in cauliflower and eggs. Season with salt and pepper, if desired.

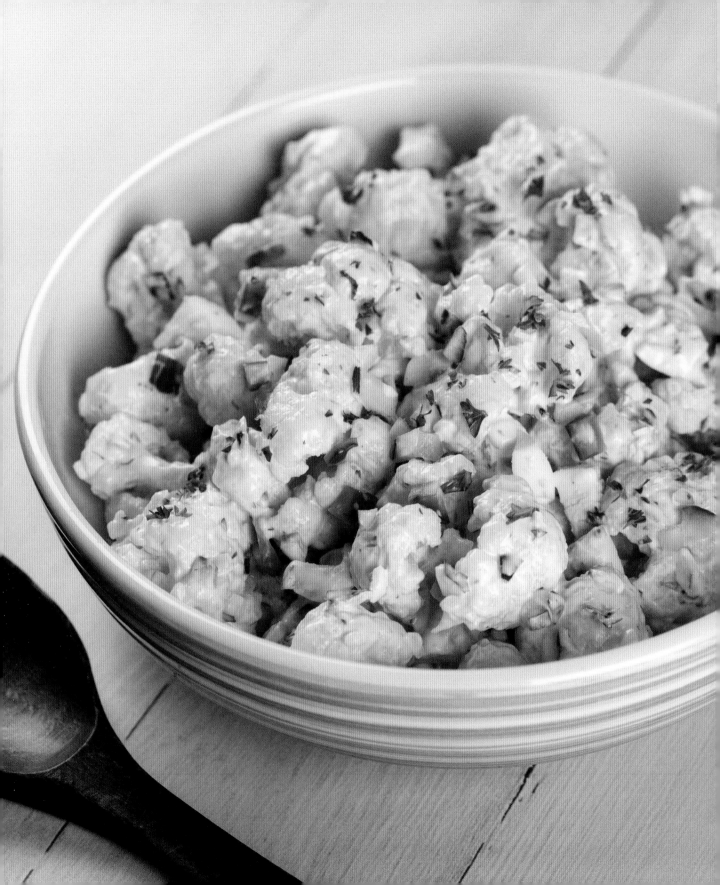

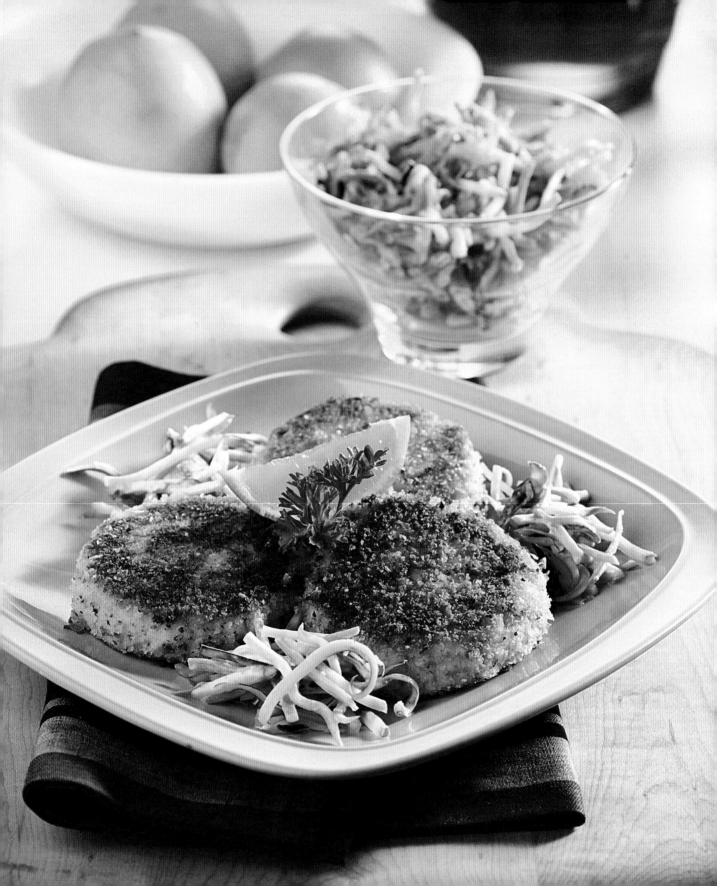

fish & seafood

Salmon and Crab Cakes

Makes 4 servings

½ **pound cooked salmon**

½ **pound cooked crabmeat***

1 **egg, lightly beaten**

1½ **tablespoons mayonnaise**

1 **tablespoon minced fresh parsley**

1 **teaspoon dried dill weed**

½ **teaspoon salt**

½ **teaspoon black pepper**

½ **teaspoon mustard**

¼ **teaspoon Worcestershire sauce**

¼ **cup plain dry bread crumbs**

Lump crabmeat works best.

1. Flake salmon and crabmeat into medium bowl. Add egg, mayonnaise, parsley, dill weed, salt, pepper, mustard and Worcestershire sauce; stir until well blended.

2. Place bread crumbs in shallow dish. Drop heaping ⅓ cup salmon mixture into bread crumbs; shape into thick patty. Repeat with remaining mixture.

3. Spray large nonstick skillet with nonstick cooking spray. Cook salmon and crab cakes, covered, over medium heat 5 to 8 minutes, turning once.

Lemon Rosemary Shrimp and Vegetable Souvlaki

Makes 4 servings

8 ounces large raw shrimp, peeled and deveined (with tails on)

1 medium zucchini, halved lengthwise and cut into ½-inch slices

½ medium red bell pepper, cut into 1-inch squares

8 green onions, trimmed and cut into 2-inch pieces

2 tablespoons extra virgin olive oil

2 tablespoons lemon juice

2 teaspoons grated lemon peel

2 medium cloves garlic, minced

½ teaspoon salt

½ teaspoon fresh rosemary

⅛ teaspoon red pepper flakes

1. Prepare grill for direct cooking. Spray grid or grill pan with nonstick cooking spray.

2. Spray four 12-inch bamboo or metal skewers with cooking spray. (If using bamboo skewers, soak in water 20 to 30 minutes before using to prevent them from burning.) Alternately thread shrimp, zucchini, bell pepper and green onions onto skewers. Spray lightly with cooking spray.

3. Combine oil, lemon juice, lemon peel, garlic, salt, rosemary and red pepper flakes in small bowl; mix well.

4. Grill skewers over high heat 2 minutes per side. Remove to large serving platter; drizzle with sauce.

Note: "Souvlaki" is the Greek word for shish kebab. Souvlaki traditionally consists of fish or meat that has been seasoned in a mixture of oil, lemon juice, and seasonings. Many souvlaki recipes, including this one, also include chunks of vegetables such as bell pepper and onion.

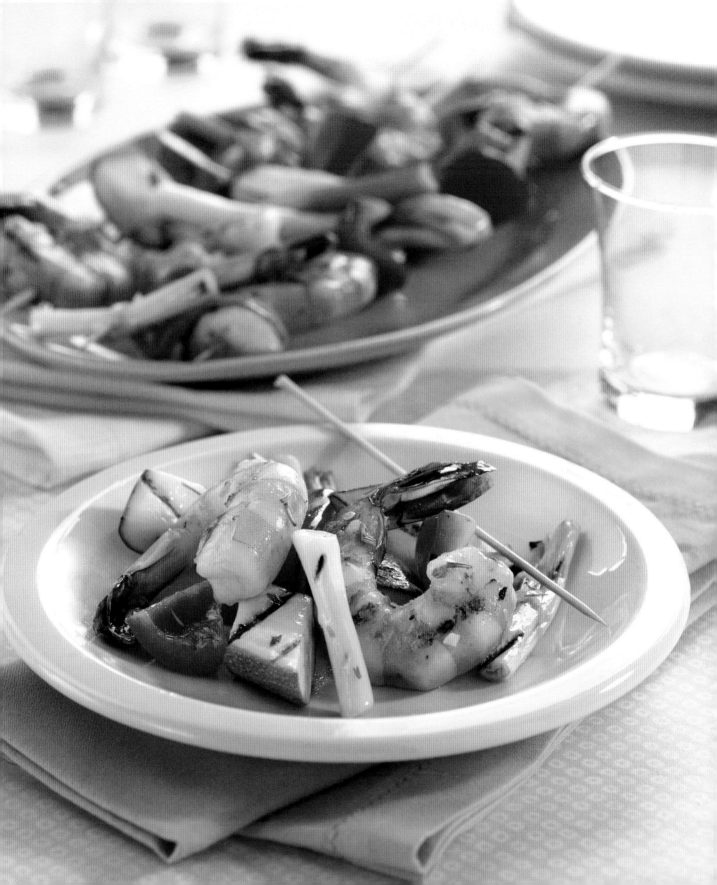

Poached Salmon with Dill-Lemon Sauce

Makes 1 serving

PER SERVING

350 **calories**
19g **total fat**
5g **carbs**
5g **net carbs**
0g **dietary fiber**
18g **protein**

- 3 **cups water**
- 1 **cup dry white wine**
  Grated peel of 1 lemon
- 3 **whole black peppercorns**
- 2 **fresh parsley sprigs**
- 1 **fresh dill sprig, plus additional for garnish**
- 1 **shallot, sliced into rings**
- 1 **salmon fillet (6 ounces), about 1 inch thick**

Dill-Lemon Sauce

- 1 **tablespoon reduced-fat mayonnaise**
- ¾ **teaspoon lemon juice**
- ½ **teaspoon canola oil**
- 1 **tablespoon milk**
- ½ **teaspoon chopped fresh dill**
  Additional fresh dill sprigs (optional)

1. Combine water, wine, lemon peel, peppercorns, parsley, 1 dill sprig and shallot in medium saucepan; bring to a simmer. Simmer gently 15 minutes. *Do not boil*.

2. Reduce heat to just below simmering. Place salmon in liquid; cook 4 to 5 minutes or until fish begins to flake when tested with fork.

3. Meanwhile for sauce, combine mayonnaise, lemon juice and oil in small bowl until blended. Whisk in milk, 1 teaspoon at a time, until well blended. Stir in chopped dill just before serving.

4. Remove salmon from liquid and place on serving plate. Top with sauce; garnish with additional dill sprigs.

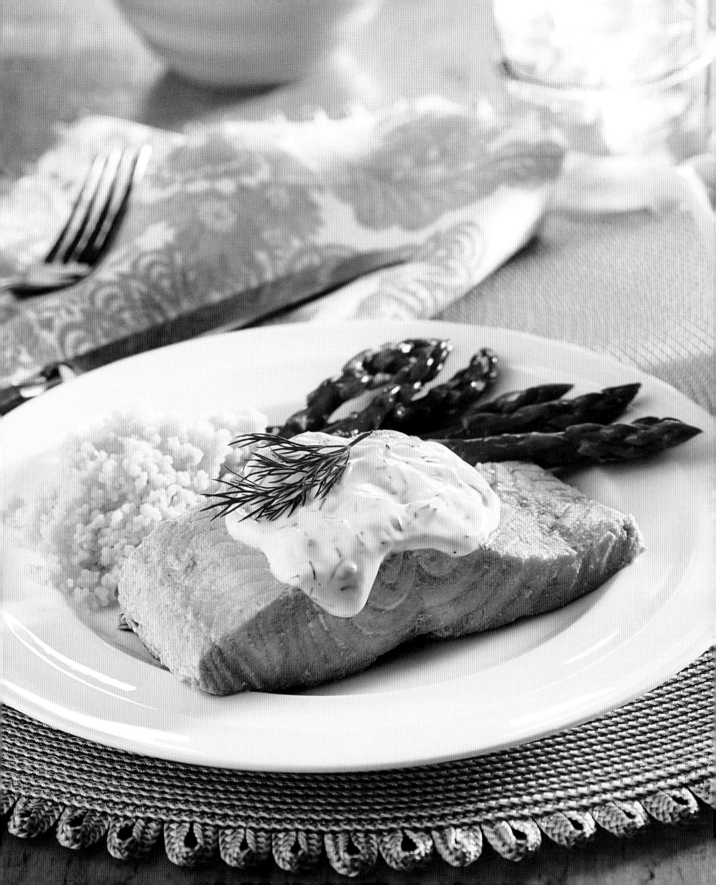

Broiled Tilapia with Mustard Cream Sauce

Makes 4 servings

4 fresh or thawed frozen tilapia fillets (about ¾ inch thick and 4 ounces each)

Black pepper

½ cup fat-free sour cream

2 tablespoons chopped fresh dill

4 teaspoons Dijon mustard

2 teaspoons lemon juice

⅛ teaspoon garlic powder

Fresh dill sprigs (optional)

1. Preheat broiler. Lightly spray rack of broiler pan with nonstick cooking spray. Place fish on rack; sprinkle with pepper.

2. Broil 4 to 5 inches from heat 5 to 8 minutes or until fish begins to flake when tested with fork. (It is not necessary to turn fish.)

3. Meanwhile, combine sour cream, chopped dill, mustard, lemon juice and garlic powder in small bowl. Serve over warm fish. Garnish with dill sprigs.

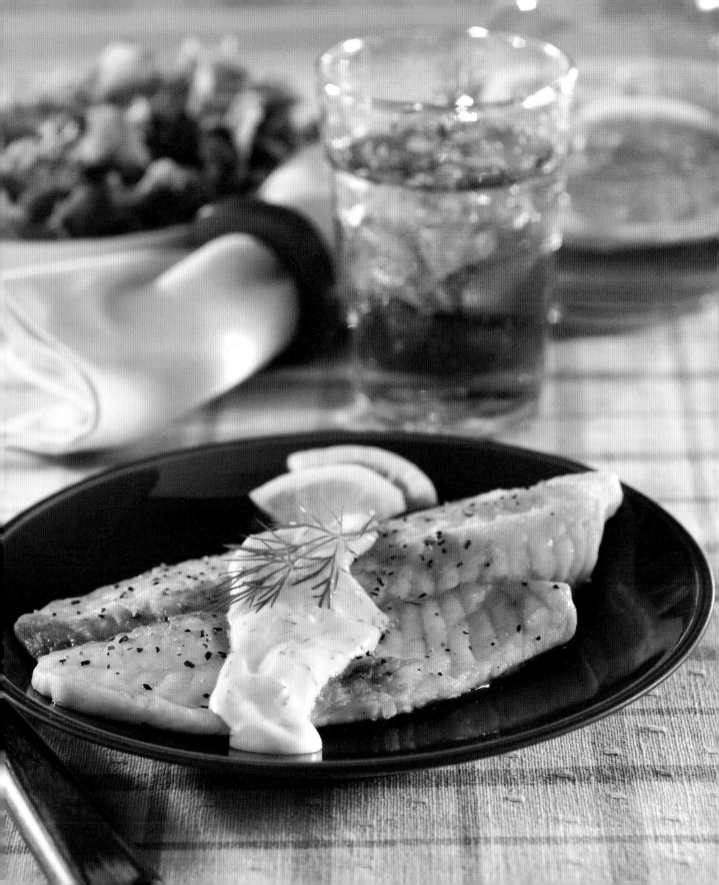

Cranberry Chutney Glazed Salmon

Makes 4 servings

PER SERVING

260 calories
15g **total fat**
6g **carbs**
6g **net carbs**
0g **dietary fiber**
23g **protein**

½ **teaspoon salt (optional)**

½ **teaspoon ground cinnamon**

¼ **teaspoon ground red pepper**

4 **skinless salmon fillets (4 ounces each)**

¼ **cup cranberry chutney**

1 **tablespoon white wine vinegar or cider vinegar**

1. Preheat broiler or prepare grill for indirect cooking. Spray rack of broiler pan with nonstick cooking spray. Combine salt, if desired, cinnamon and red pepper in small bowl; rub over salmon. Combine chutney and vinegar in small bowl; brush about 1 tablespoon over each salmon fillet.

2. Broil salmon 5 to 6 inches from heat source or grill over medium-hot coals on covered grill 4 to 6 minutes or until opaque in center.

Variation: If cranberry chutney is not available, substitute mango chutney. Chop any large pieces of mango.

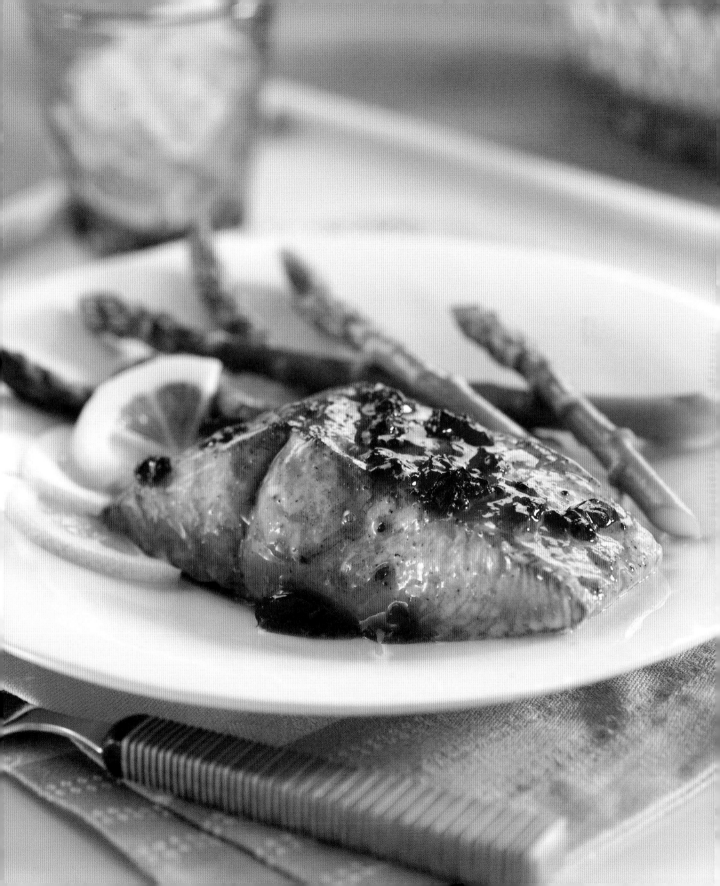

Shrimp and Veggie Skillet Toss

Makes 4 servings

PER SERVING

110 **calories**
4.5g **total fat**
10g **carbs**
8g **net carbs**
2g **dietary fiber**
11g **protein**

¼ cup reduced-sodium soy sauce

2 tablespoons lime juice

1 tablespoon sesame oil

1 teaspoon grated fresh ginger

⅛ teaspoon red pepper flakes

32 medium raw shrimp (about 8 ounces total), peeled, deveined, rinsed and patted dry (with tails on)

2 medium zucchini, cut in half lengthwise and thinly sliced

6 green onions, trimmed and halved lengthwise

12 grape tomatoes

1. Whisk soy sauce, lime juice, oil, ginger and red pepper flakes in small bowl; set aside.

2. Spray large nonstick skillet with nonstick cooking spray; heat over medium-high heat. Add shrimp; cook and stir 3 minutes or until shrimp are opaque. Remove from skillet.

3. Spray same skillet with cooking spray. Add zucchini; cook and stir 4 to 6 minutes or just until crisp-tender. Add green onions and tomatoes; cook 1 to 2 minutes. Add shrimp, cook 1 minute. Transfer to large bowl.

4. Add soy sauce mixture to skillet; bring to a boil. Remove from heat. Stir in shrimp and vegetables; gently toss.

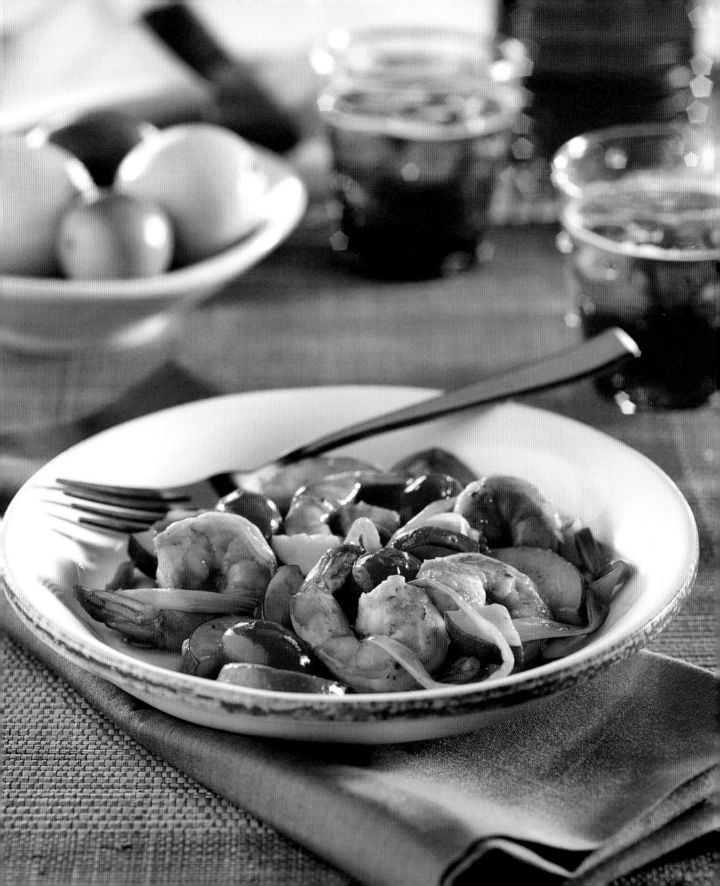

Mustard-Grilled Red Snapper

Makes 4 servings

PER SERVING

200 calories
2.5g **total fat**
0g **carbs**
0g **net carbs**
0g **dietary fiber**
35g **protein**

½ cup Dijon mustard

1 tablespoon red wine vinegar

1 teaspoon ground red pepper

4 red snapper fillets (about 6 ounces each)

Fresh parsley sprigs and red peppercorns (optional)

1. Prepare grill for direct cooking. Spray grid with nonstick cooking spray.

2. Combine mustard, vinegar and red pepper in small bowl; mix well. Coat fish thoroughly with mustard mixture.

3. Grill fish, covered, over medium-high heat 8 minutes or until fish begins to flake easily when tested with fork, turning halfway through grilling time. Garnish with parsley sprigs and red peppercorns.

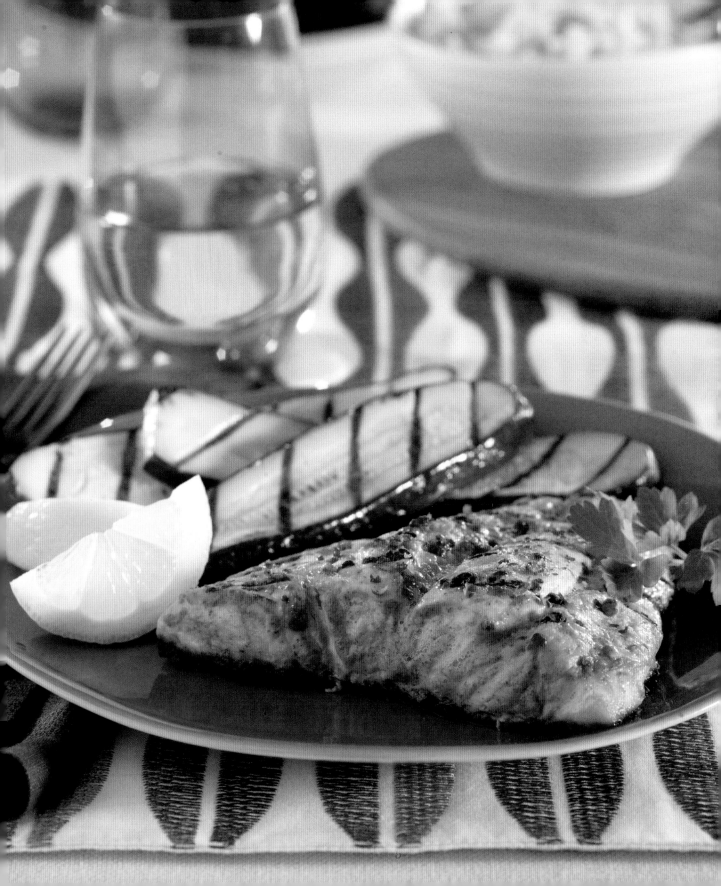

Baked Fish with Tomatoes & Herbs

Makes 4 servings

PER SERVING

150 **calories**
4g **total fat**
4g **carbs**
3g **net carbs**
1g **dietary fiber**
24g **protein**

- 4 **lean white fish fillets (about 1 pound), such as orange roughy or sole**
- 2 **tablespoons plus 2 teaspoons lemon juice, divided**
- ½ **teaspoon paprika**
- 1 **cup finely chopped seeded tomatoes**
- 2 **tablespoons capers, rinsed and drained**
- 2 **tablespoons finely chopped fresh parsley**
- 1½ **teaspoons dried basil**
- 2 **teaspoons olive oil**
- ¼ **teaspoon salt**

1. Preheat oven to 350°F. Coat 12×8-inch glass baking dish with nonstick cooking spray.

2. Arrange fish fillets in dish. Drizzle 2 tablespoons lemon juice over fillets; sprinkle with paprika. Cover with foil; bake 18 minutes or until opaque in center and flakes easily when tested with fork.

3. Meanwhile, in medium saucepan, combine tomatoes, capers, parsley, remaining 2 teaspoons lemon juice, basil, oil and salt. Five minutes before fish is done, place saucepan over high heat. Bring to a boil. Reduce heat and simmer 2 minutes or until hot. Remove from heat.

4. Serve fish topped with tomato mixture.

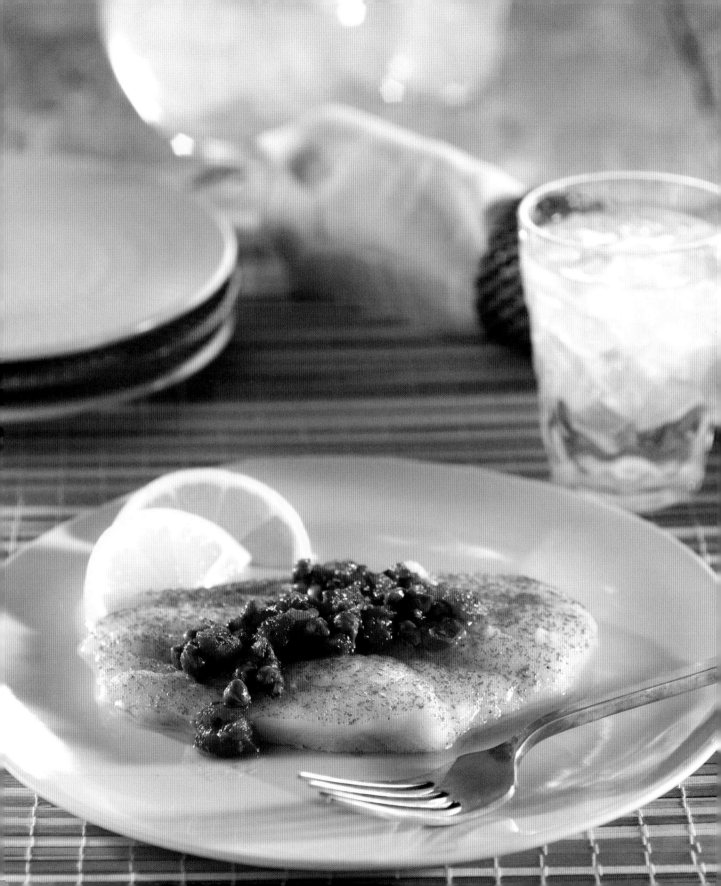

Skillet Fish with Lemon Tarragon "Butter"

Makes 2 servings

- 2 **teaspoons butter**
- 4 **teaspoons lemon juice, divided**
- ½ **teaspoon grated lemon peel**
- ¼ **teaspoon prepared mustard**
- ¼ **teaspoon dried tarragon**
- ⅛ **teaspoon salt**
- 2 **lean white fish fillets (4 ounces each),* rinsed and patted dry**
- ¼ **teaspoon paprika**

Cod, orange roughy, flounder, haddock, halibut and sole can be used.

1. Combine butter, 2 teaspoons lemon juice, lemon peel, mustard, tarragon and salt in small bowl; mix well with fork.

2. Spray 12-inch nonstick skillet with nonstick cooking spray; heat over medium heat. Drizzle fish with remaining 2 teaspoons lemon juice; sprinkle one side of each fillet with paprika.

3. Place fish in skillet, paprika side down; cook 3 minutes. Gently turn and cook 3 minutes longer or until fish is opaque in center and begins to flake when tested with fork. Top with butter mixture.

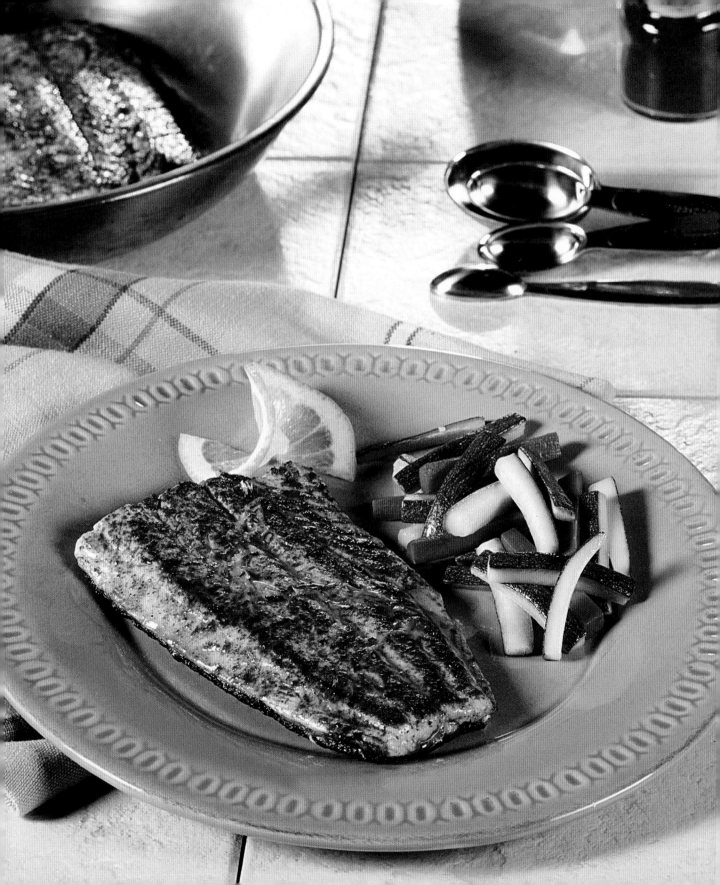

Red Snapper Scampi

Makes 4 servings

¼ **cup (½ stick) butter or margarine, softened**

1 **tablespoon dry white wine**

1½ **teaspoons minced garlic**

½ **teaspoon grated lemon peel**

⅛ **teaspoon black pepper**

1½ **pounds red snapper, orange roughy or grouper fillets (4 to 5 ounces each)**

1. Preheat oven to 450°F. Combine butter, wine, garlic, lemon peel and pepper in small bowl until blended.

2. Place fish in foil-lined shallow baking pan. Top with seasoned butter. Bake 10 to 12 minutes or until fish just begins to flake when tested with fork.

Tip: Serve fish with mixed salad greens, if desired. Or, add sliced carrots, zucchini and bell pepper cut into matchstick-size strips to the baking pan with the fish for an easy vegetable side dish.

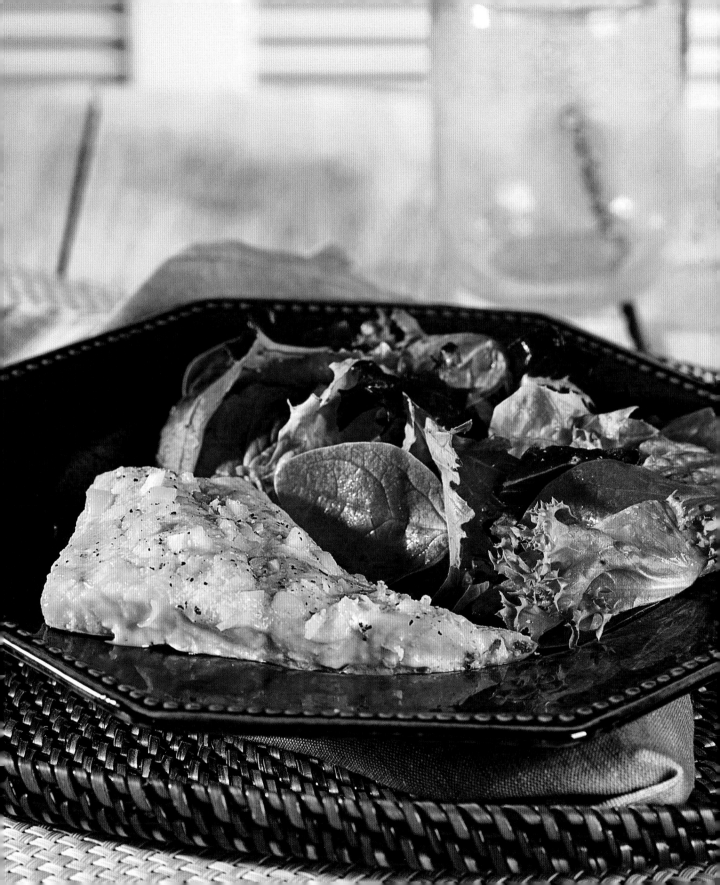

Elegant Shrimp Scampi

Makes 8 servings

PER SERVING

150 **calories**
10g **total fat**
3g **carbs**
3g **net carbs**
0g **dietary fiber**
12g **protein**

¼ cup (½ stick) plus 2 tablespoons butter

6 to 8 cloves garlic, minced

1½ pounds large raw shrimp (about 16), peeled and deveined (with tails on)

6 green onions, thinly sliced

¼ cup dry white wine or chicken broth

Juice of 1 lemon (about 2 tablespoons)

¼ cup chopped fresh parsley

Salt and black pepper

Lemon slices (optional)

1. Clarify butter by melting it in small saucepan over low heat. ***Do not stir.*** Skim off white foam that forms on top. Strain clarified butter through cheesecloth into glass measuring cup to yield ⅓ cup. Discard cheesecloth and milky residue at bottom of pan.

2. Heat clarified butter in large skillet over medium heat. Add garlic; cook and stir 1 to 2 minutes or until softened but not browned.

3. Add shrimp, green onions, wine and lemon juice; cook and stir 3 to 4 minutes or until shrimp are pink and opaque. ***Do not overcook.***

4. Stir in parsley and season with salt and pepper. Garnish with lemon slices.

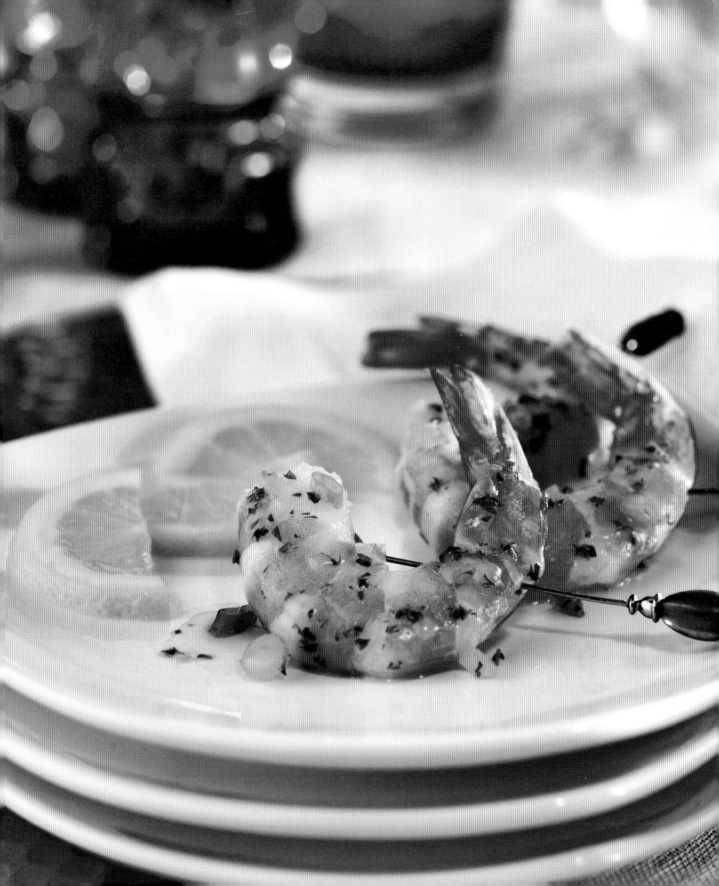

Soy-Marinated Salmon

Makes 4 servings

PER SERVING

310 calories
19g **total fat**
2g **carbs**
2g **net carbs**
0g **dietary fiber**
31g **protein**

¼ **cup soy sauce**

⅛ **cup lime juice**

1 **tablespoon grated fresh ginger**

1 **tablespoon minced garlic**

¼ **teaspoon black pepper**

4 **salmon fillets (5 to 6 ounces each)**

2 **tablespoons minced green onion**

1. Combine soy sauce, lime juice, ginger, garlic and pepper in medium bowl; mix well. Reserve ¼ cup mixture for serving; set aside. Place salmon in large resealable food storage bag. Pour remaining mixture over salmon; seal bag and turn to coat. Marinate in refrigerator 2 to 4 hours, turning occasionally.

2. Prepare grill or preheat broiler. Remove salmon from marinade; discard marinade.

3. Grill or broil salmon 10 minutes or until fish begins to flake when tested with fork. (To broil, place salmon on foil-lined baking sheet sprayed with nonstick cooking spray.) Brush with some of reserved marinade mixture; sprinkle with green onion.

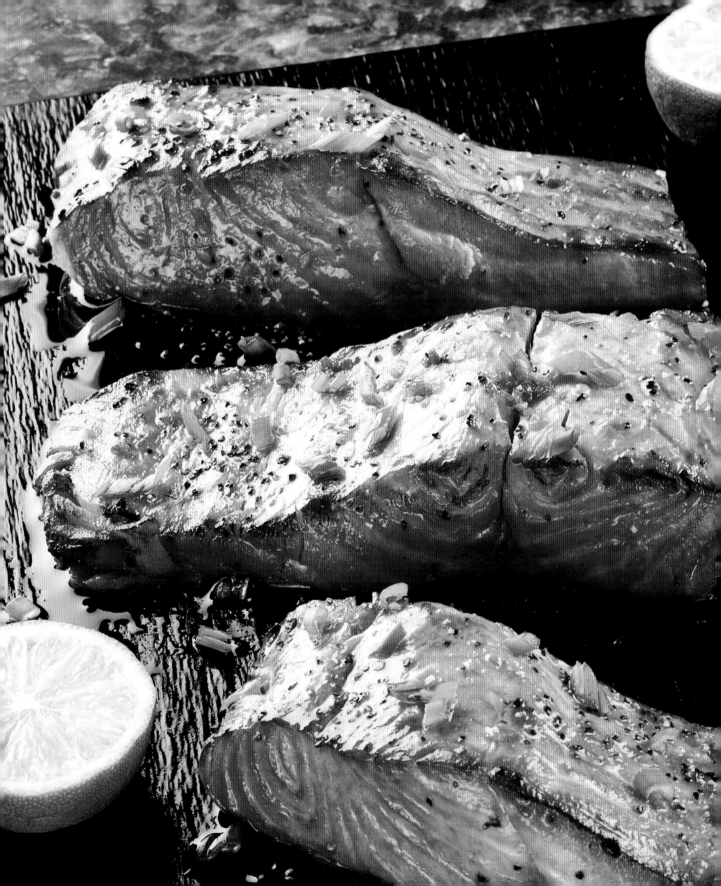

Salmon with Bok Choy

Makes 4 servings

PER SERVING

280 **calories**
15g **total fat**
9g **carbs**
8g **net carbs**
1g **dietary fiber**
25g **protein**

- **4** skinless salmon fillets (4 ounces each)
- **3** tablespoons finely chopped fresh ginger
- **2** cloves garlic, minced
- **½** cup reduced-sodium vegetable broth
- **3** tablespoons unseasoned rice vinegar
- **1** tablespoon reduced-sodium soy sauce
- **6** cups chopped bok choy
- **1** teaspoon hoisin sauce
- **¼** cup sliced green onions

Slow Cooker Directions

1. Spray slow cooker with nonstick cooking spray. Arrange salmon in slow cooker; spread ginger and garlic evenly over salmon. Pour broth, vinegar and soy sauce over salmon. Cover; cook on LOW 1½ hours.

2. Add bok choy to slow cooker; cover and cook 30 minutes or until crisp-tender and salmon flakes easily when tested with fork.

3. Remove salmon from slow cooker; arrange on four plates. Stir hoisin sauce into liquid in slow cooker.

4. Spoon sauce evenly over salmon. Top with green onions. Serve with bok choy.

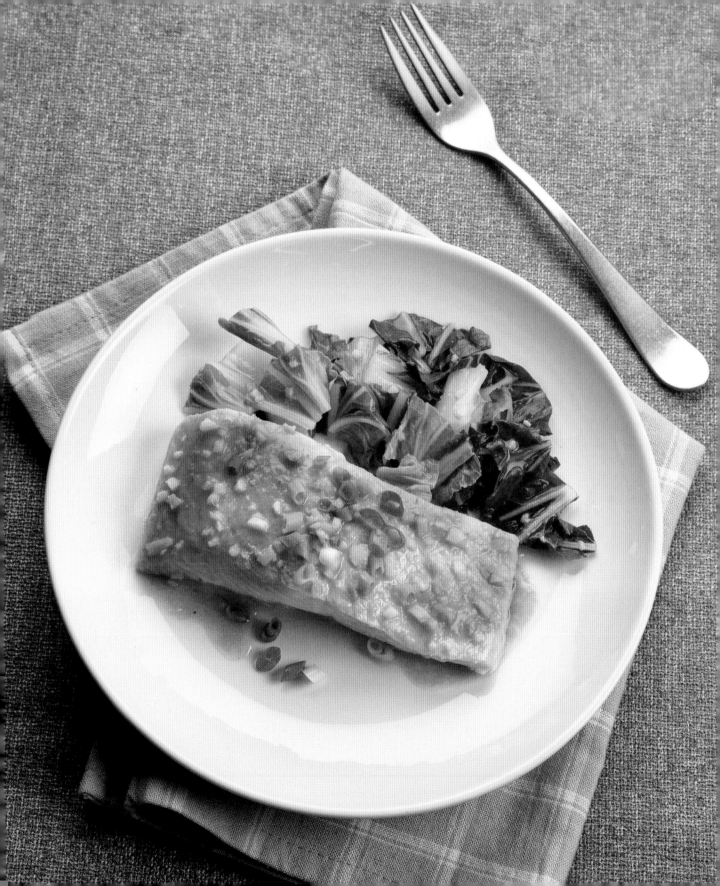

Grilled Five-Spice Fish with Garlic Spinach

Makes 4 servings

1½ teaspoons grated lime peel

3 tablespoons fresh lime juice

4 teaspoons minced fresh ginger

½ to 1 teaspoon Chinese five-spice powder

½ teaspoon salt

⅛ teaspoon black pepper

2 teaspoons vegetable oil, divided

1 pound salmon steaks

8 ounces fresh baby spinach leaves (about 8 cups lightly packed), washed

2 cloves garlic, minced

1. Combine lime peel, lime juice, ginger, five-spice powder, salt, pepper and 1 teaspoon oil in 2-quart baking dish. Add salmon; turn to coat. Cover; refrigerate 2 to 3 hours.

2. Combine spinach, garlic and remaining 1 teaspoon oil in 3-quart microwavable dish; toss. Cover; microwave on HIGH 2 minutes or until spinach is wilted. Drain; keep warm.

3. Meanwhile, prepare grill for direct cooking over medium-high heat. Spray with nonstick cooking spray.

4. Remove salmon from marinade and place on grid. Brush salmon with marinade. Grill salmon, covered, 4 minutes. Turn salmon; brush with marinade and grill 4 minutes or until fish just begins to flake when tested with fork. Discard remaining marinade.

5. Serve fish over bed of spinach.

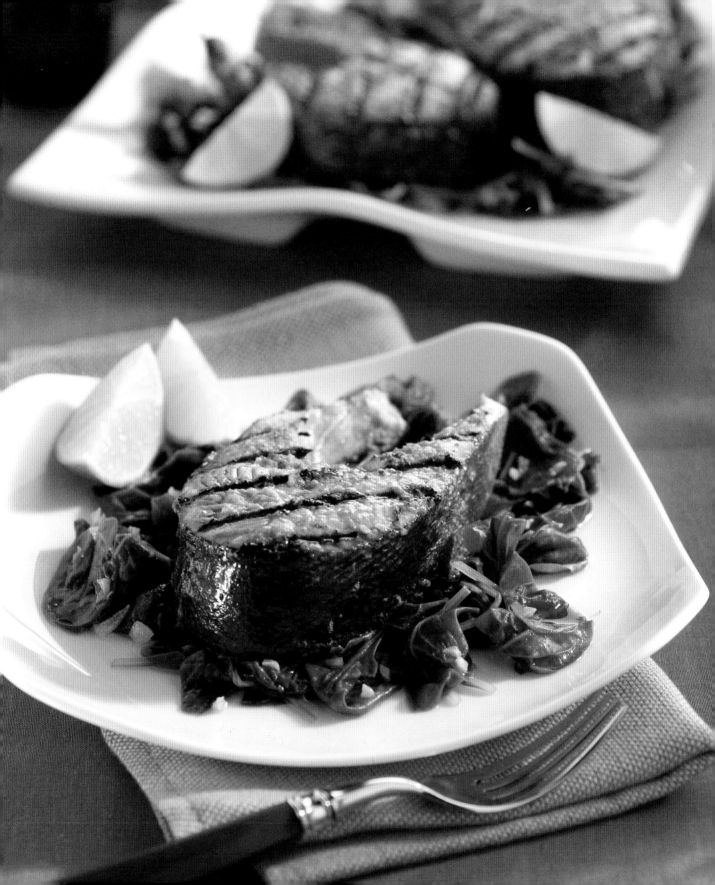

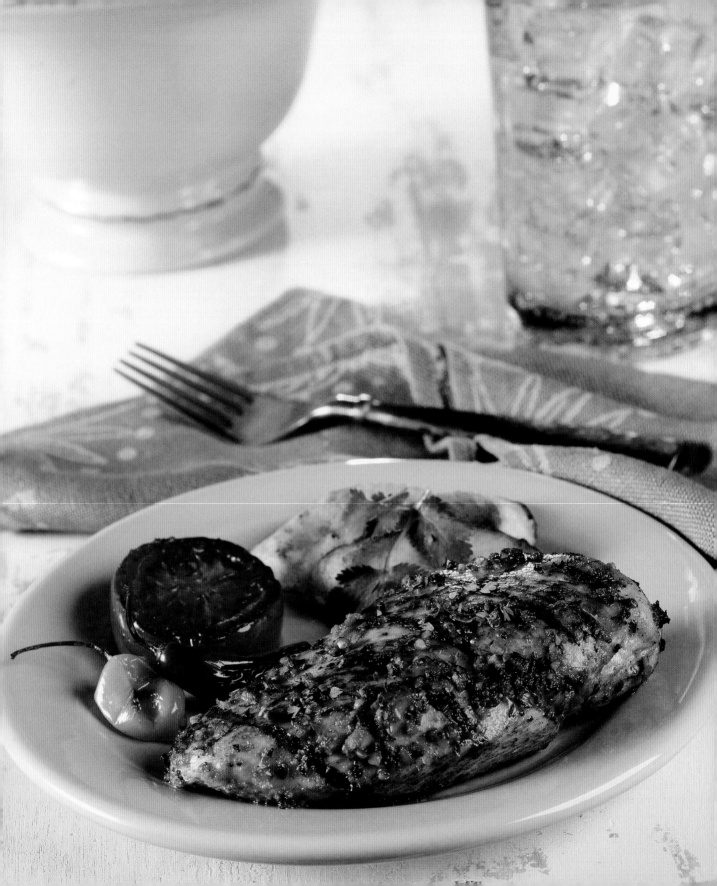

chicken & turkey

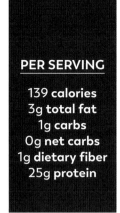

Grilled Chicken Adobo

Makes 4 servings

½ **cup chopped onion**

⅓ **cup lime juice**

6 **cloves garlic, coarsely chopped**

1 **teaspoon ground cumin**

1 **teaspoon dried oregano**

½ **teaspoon dried thyme**

¼ **teaspoon ground red pepper**

4 **boneless skinless chicken breasts (about 1 pound total)**

3 **tablespoons chopped fresh cilantro (optional)**

1. Combine onion, lime juice and garlic in food processor. Process until onion is finely minced. Transfer to large resealable food storage bag. Add cumin, oregano, thyme and red pepper; knead bag until blended. Place chicken in bag; press out air and seal. Turn to coat chicken with marinade. Refrigerate 30 minutes or up to 4 hours, turning occasionally.

2. Prepare grill for direct cooking. Spray grid with nonstick cooking spray. Remove chicken from marinade; discard marinade. Place chicken on grid. Grill 5 to 7 minutes on each side over medium heat or until chicken is no longer pink in center. Transfer to clean serving platter and garnish with cilantro, if desired.

Quick Orange Chicken

Makes 4 servings

PER SERVING

157 **calories**
1g **total fat**
8g **carbs**
7g **net carbs**
1g **dietary fiber**
27g **protein**

- 2 tablespoons frozen orange juice concentrate
- 1 tablespoon no-sugar-added orange marmalade
- 1 teaspoon Dijon mustard
- ¼ teaspoon salt
- 4 boneless skinless chicken breasts (about 1 pound)
- ½ cup fresh orange sections
- 2 tablespoons chopped fresh parsley

Microwave Directions

1. For sauce, combine juice concentrate, marmalade, mustard and salt in 8-inch shallow microwavable dish until juice concentrate is thawed.

2. Add chicken, coating both sides with sauce. Arrange chicken around edge of dish without overlapping. Cover with vented plastic wrap. Microwave on HIGH 3 minutes; turn chicken over. Microwave on MEDIUM-HIGH (70%) 4 minutes or until chicken is no longer pink in center.

3. Remove chicken to serving plate. Microwave remaining sauce on HIGH 2 to 3 minutes or until slightly thickened.

4. To serve, spoon sauce over chicken; top with orange sections and parsley.

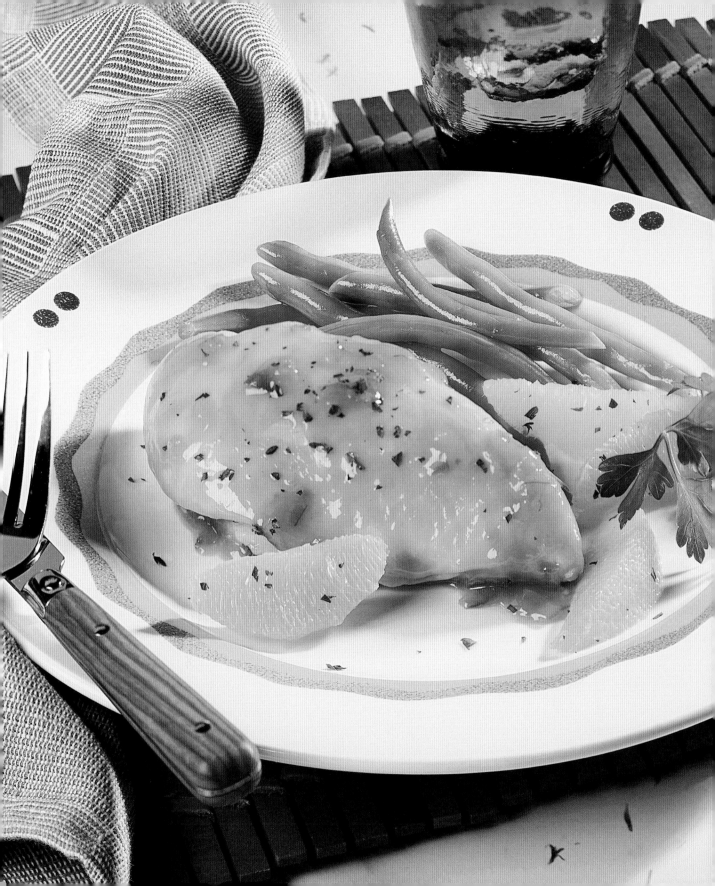

Turkey Meatballs with Spaghetti Squash

Makes 6 servings

- 1 **egg**
- 1 **pound ground turkey**
- ½ **cup finely chopped onion**
- ¼ **cup almond flour**
- 2 **tablespoons chopped fresh parsley**
- 1¼ **teaspoons salt, divided**
- 1 **teaspoon garlic powder**
- ¾ **teaspoon dried thyme**
- ¼ **teaspoon fennel seeds**
- ¼ **teaspoon black pepper**
- ⅛ **teaspoon red pepper flakes**
- 1 **(12- to 16-ounce) spaghetti squash**
- ¼ **cup water**
- 1 **can (about 14 ounces) crushed tomatoes**
- ¾ **cup chicken broth**
- ⅓ **cup finely chopped green onions**
- ½ **teaspoon dried basil**
- ½ **teaspoon dried oregano**

1. Preheat broiler. Line baking sheet with foil; spray foil with nonstick cooking spray. Beat egg in large bowl. Add turkey, onion, almond flour, parsley, 1 teaspoon salt, garlic powder, thyme, fennel seeds, black pepper and red pepper flakes; mix gently until blended. Shape mixture into meatballs; place on prepared baking sheet.

2. Broil meatballs 4 to 5 minutes or until tops are browned. Turn meatballs; broil 4 minutes.

3. Split squash in half and remove seeds. Place in glass baking dish, cut sides down; add water. Microwave on HIGH 10 to 12 minutes or until fork-tender. Set aside to cool.

4. Meanwhile, combine tomatoes, broth, green onions, basil, oregano and remaining ¼ teaspoon salt in large skillet; bring to a simmer over medium heat. Add meatballs; stir to coat. Reduce heat to medium-low; cook 10 minutes.

5. Scrape squash into strands onto serving plate. Top with meatballs and sauce.

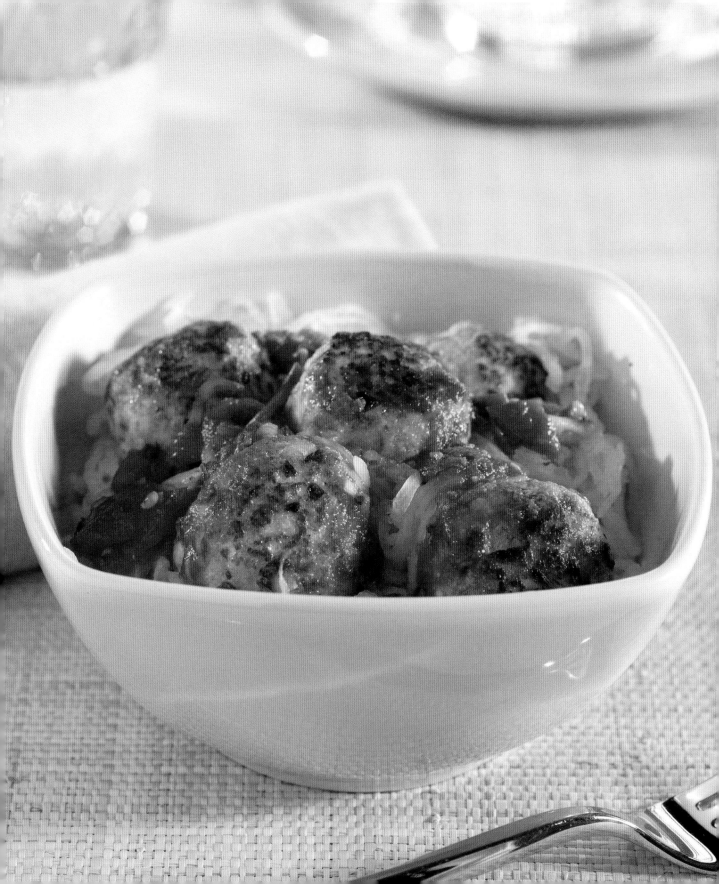

Sheet Pan Chicken and Sausage Supper

Makes 6 servings

⅓ **cup olive oil**

2 **tablespoons balsamic vinegar**

1 **teaspoon salt**

1 **teaspoon garlic powder**

½ **teaspoon black pepper**

¼ **teaspoon red pepper flakes**

3 **pounds bone-in chicken thighs and drumsticks**

1 **pound uncooked sweet Italian sausage (4 to 5 links), cut diagonally into 2-inch pieces**

6 **to 8 small red onions (about 1½ pounds), each cut into 6 wedges**

3½ **cups broccoli florets**

1. Preheat oven to 425°F. Line baking sheet with foil, if desired.

2. Whisk oil, vinegar, salt, garlic powder, black pepper and red pepper flakes in small bowl until well blended. Combine chicken, sausage and onions on prepared baking sheet. Drizzle with oil mixture; toss until well coated. Spread meat and onions in single layer (chicken thighs should be skin side up).

3. Bake 30 minutes. Add broccoli to baking sheet; stir to coat broccoli with pan juices and turn sausage. Bake 30 minutes or until broccoli is beginning to brown and chicken is cooked through (165°F).

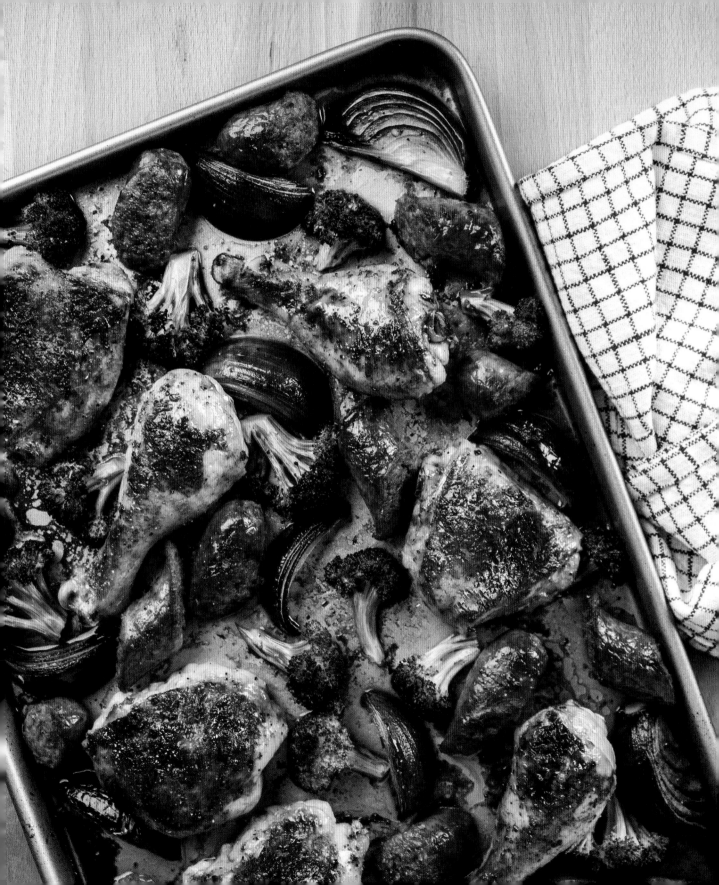

Chicken with Artichokes

Makes 4 servings

PER SERVING

240 calories
11g **total fat**
8g **carbs**
3g **net carbs**
5g **dietary fiber**
28g **protein**

½ **teaspoon salt, divided**

⅛ **teaspoon black pepper**

2 **whole broiler-fryer chicken breasts, halved, boned, skinned**

2 **tablespoons olive oil**

½ **medium red pepper, cut into thin strips**

2 **cloves garlic, minced**

1 **package (9 ounces) frozen artichoke hearts**

¾ **cup chicken broth**

1 **tablespoon lemon juice**

½ **teaspoon dried marjoram**

1. Sprinkle ¼ teaspoon salt and pepper over chicken. Heat oil in large skillet over medium-high heat. Add red pepper strips; cook and stir 2 to 3 minutes or until tender. Remove to small bowl.

2. Add chicken to skillet; cook about 6 minutes, turning once, or until browned on both sides. Add garlic; cook 1 minute. Add artichoke hearts, broth, lemon juice, marjoram and remaining ¼ teaspoon salt. Bring to a boil. Reduce heat; cover and cook about 10 minutes or until chicken and artichokes are fork-tender. Top each serving with red pepper strips.

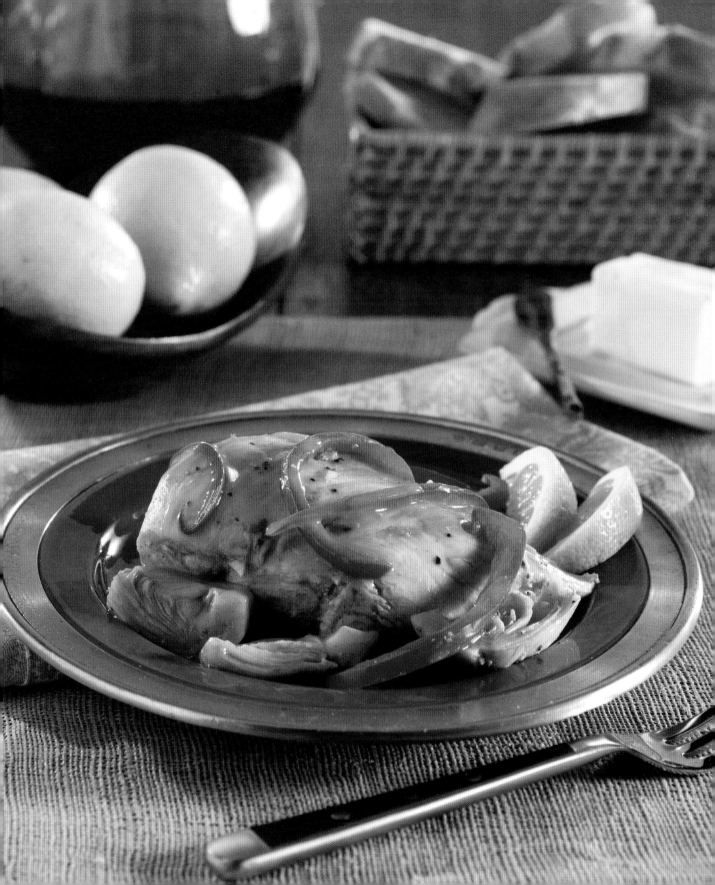

Turkey and Veggie Meatballs with Fennel

Makes 6 servings

- 1 **pound lean ground turkey**
- ½ **cup finely chopped green onions**
- ½ **cup finely chopped green bell pepper**
- ⅓ **cup almond flour**
- 2 **tablespoons whipping cream**
- ¼ **cup shredded carrot**
- ¼ **cup grated Parmesan cheese**
- 2 **egg whites**
- 2 **cloves garlic, minced**
- ½ **teaspoon Italian seasoning**
- ¼ **teaspoon fennel seeds**
- ¼ **teaspoon salt**
- ⅛ **teaspoon red pepper flakes (optional)**
- 1 **teaspoon extra virgin olive oil**

1. Combine all ingredients except oil in large bowl; mix well. Shape into 36 (1-inch) balls.

2. Heat oil in large nonstick skillet over medium-high heat. Add meatballs; cook 11 minutes or until no longer pink in center, turning frequently. Use fork and spoon for easy turning. Serve immediately or cool and freeze.*

To freeze, cool completely and place in gallon-size resealable food storage bag. Release any excess air from bag and seal. Freeze bag flat for easier storage and faster thawing. This will also allow you to remove as many meatballs as needed without them sticking together. To reheat, place meatballs in a 12×8-inch microwavable dish and cook on HIGH 20 to 30 seconds or until hot.

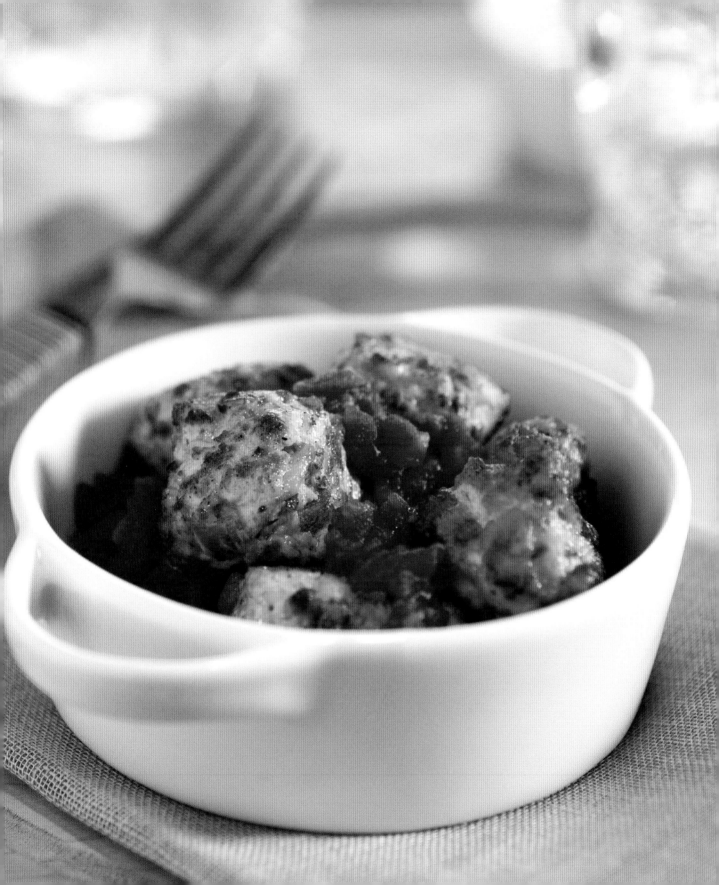

Turkey Taco Bowls

Makes 4 servings

1 tablespoon chili powder

1 teaspoon paprika

1 teaspoon ground cumin

½ teaspoon dried oregano

½ teaspoon salt

¼ teaspoon garlic powder

¼ teaspoon onion powder

1 pound ground turkey

¾ cup water

1 bag (10 ounces) frozen cauliflower rice

2 cups shredded red cabbage

2 green onions, finely chopped

1 avocado, thinly sliced

2 plum tomatoes, diced

Minced fresh cilantro, sour cream and crumbled cotija cheese

1. Combine chili powder, paprika, cumin, oregano, salt, garlic powder and onion powder in small bowl.

2. Cook turkey in large nonstick skillet over medium-high heat 6 to 8 minutes or until no longer pink, stirring to break up meat. Stir in spice mix and water; bring to a boil. Reduce heat to medium-low; simmer 5 minutes, stirring occasionally. Set aside.

3. Heat cauliflower rice according to package directions. Divide among four bowls. Add turkey, cabbage, green onions, avocado and tomatoes. Serve with cilantro, sour cream and cotija cheese.

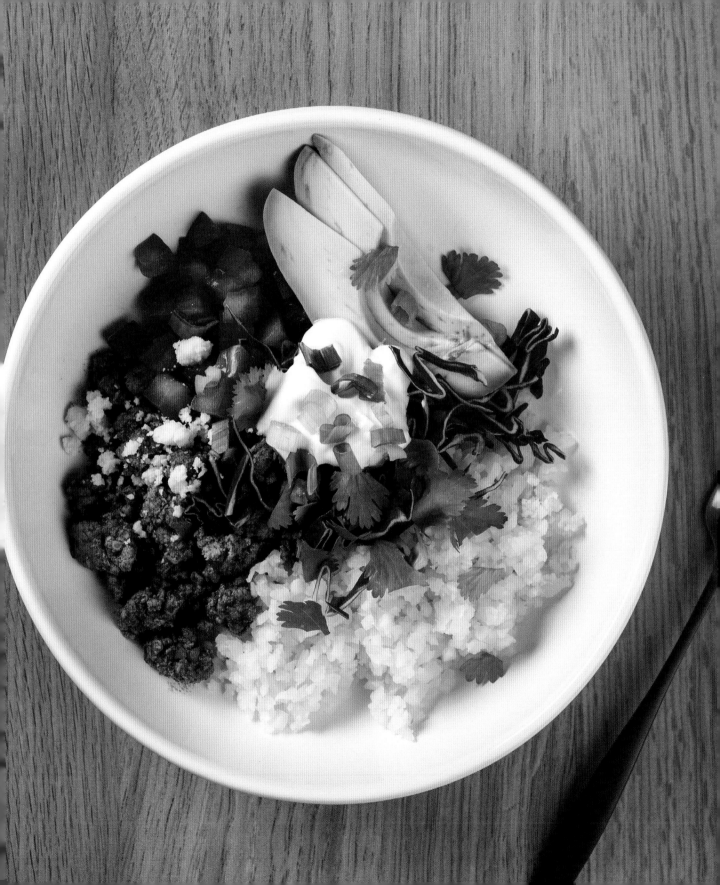

Greek Chicken Burgers with Cucumber Yogurt Sauce

Makes 4 servings

½ cup plus 2 tablespoons plain nonfat Greek yogurt

½ medium cucumber, peeled, seeded and finely chopped

Juice of ½ lemon

3 cloves garlic, minced, divided

2 teaspoons finely chopped fresh mint *or* ½ teaspoon dried mint

⅛ teaspoon salt

⅛ teaspoon ground white pepper

1 pound ground chicken breast

3 ounces reduced-fat crumbled feta cheese

4 large kalamata olives, rinsed, patted dry and minced

1 egg

½ to 1 teaspoon dried oregano

¼ teaspoon black pepper

Mixed baby lettuce (optional)

Fresh mint leaves (optional)

1. Combine yogurt, cucumber, lemon juice, 2 cloves garlic, 2 teaspoons chopped mint, salt and white pepper in medium bowl; mix well. Cover and refrigerate until ready to serve.

2. Combine chicken, cheese, olives, egg, oregano, black pepper and remaining 1 clove garlic in large bowl; mix well. Shape mixture into four patties.

3. Spray grill pan with nonstick cooking spray; heat over medium-high heat. Grill patties 5 to 7 minutes per side or until cooked through (165°F).

4. Serve burgers with sauce and mixed greens, if desired. Garnish with mint leaves.

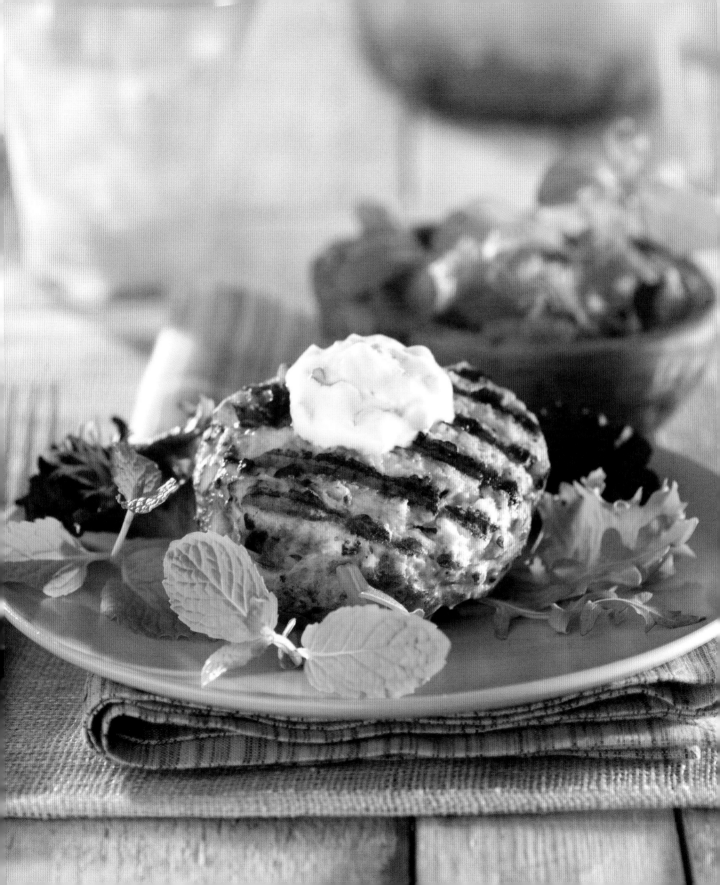

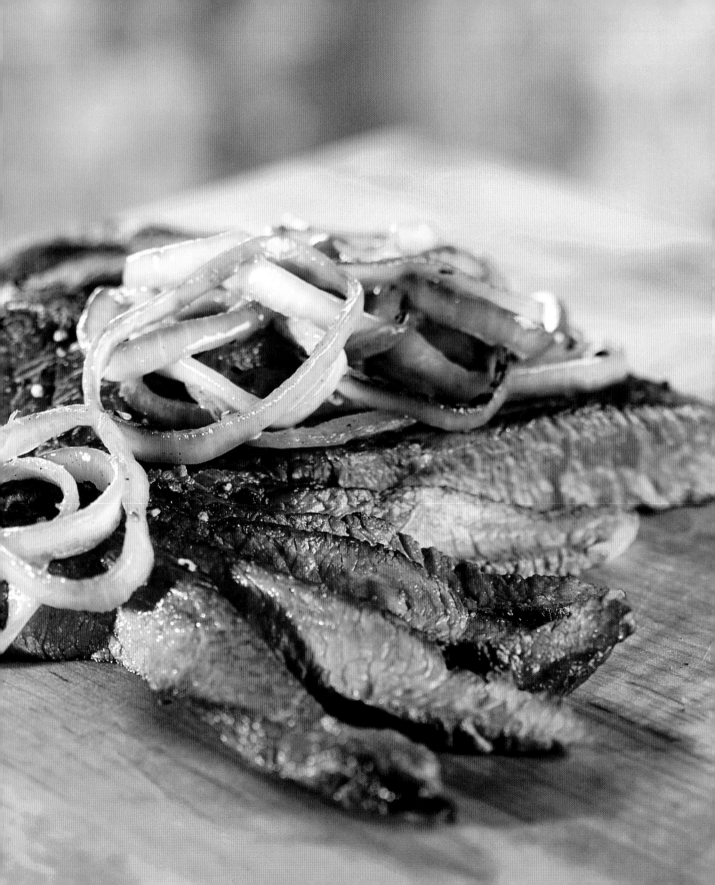

beef, pork & lamb

Sirloin with Sweet Caramelized Onions

Makes 4 servings

1 **medium onion, very thinly sliced**

1 **boneless beef top sirloin steak (about 1 pound)**

¼ **cup water**

2 **tablespoons Worcestershire sauce**

1 **tablespoon sugar**

1. Lightly coat 12-inch skillet with nonstick cooking spray; heat over high heat. Add onion; cook and stir 4 minutes or until browned. Remove from skillet and set aside. Wipe out skillet with paper towel.

2. Coat same skillet with cooking spray; heat over high heat. Add beef; cook 10 to 13 minutes for medium rare to medium, turning once. Remove from heat and transfer steak to cutting board; let stand 3 minutes before slicing.

3. Meanwhile, return skillet to high heat; add onion, water, Worcestershire sauce and sugar. Cook 30 to 45 seconds or until most liquid has evaporated.

4. Thinly slice beef on the diagonal; serve with onions.

Pork Tenderloin with Avocado-Tomatillo Salsa

Makes 4 servings

PER SERVING

174 calories
6g **total fat**
4g **carbs**
2g **net carbs**
2g **dietary fiber**
25g **protein**

1½   teaspoons chili powder

½   teaspoon ground cumin

1   pound pork tenderloin

1   teaspoon extra virgin olive oil

Salsa

2   medium tomatillos, husked*
     and diced

½   ripe medium avocado, diced

1   jalapeño pepper,** seeded and
     finely chopped

1   clove garlic, minced

2   tablespoons finely chopped red
     onion

1   tablespoon lime juice

1   to 2 tablespoons chopped
     fresh cilantro

⅛   teaspoon salt

4   lime wedges (optional)

Remove the husk by pulling from the bottom to where it attaches at the stem. Wash before using.

**Jalapeño peppers can sting and irritate the skin, so wear rubber gloves when handling and do not touch your eyes.*

1. Preheat oven to 425°F. Combine chili powder and cumin in small bowl. Sprinkle evenly on pork, pressing to allow spices to adhere.

2. Heat oil in large nonstick skillet over medium-high heat until hot. Add pork and cook 3 minutes. Turn; cook 2 to 3 minutes longer or until richly browned. Place on foil-lined baking sheet; bake 20 to 25 minutes or until barely pink in center (about 165°F). Remove from oven and let stand 5 minutes before slicing.

3. Combine salsa ingredients in small bowl and toss gently to blend. Serve with pork slices and additional lime wedges, if desired.

Tip: Choose firm tomatillos with dry husks that are not too ragged. Store in a paper bag in refrigerator for up to 1 month.

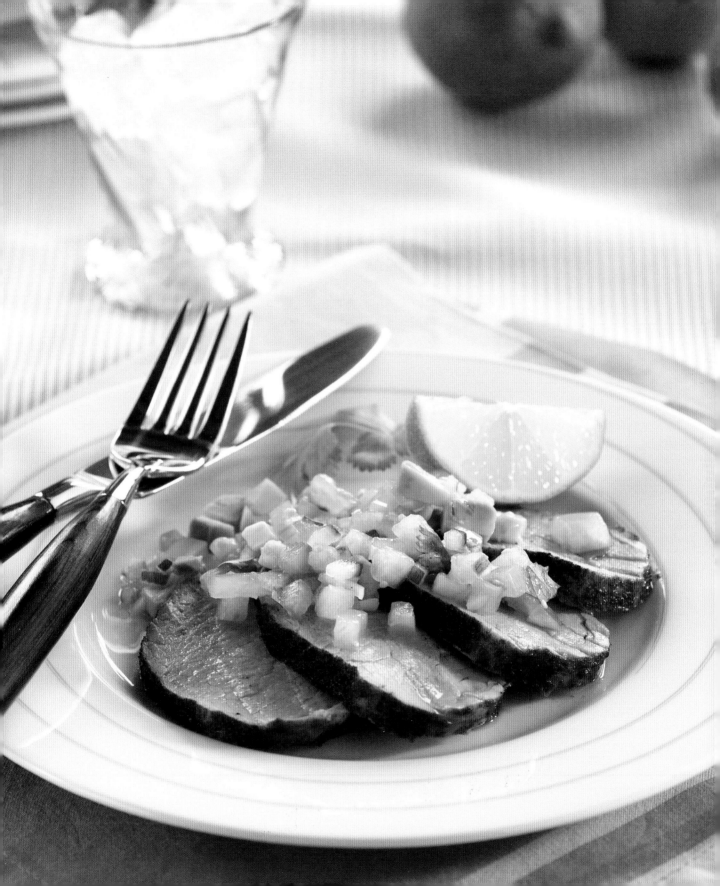

Zesty Skillet Pork Chops

Makes 4 servings

PER SERVING

172 **calories**
7g **total fat**
9g **carbs**
6g **net carbs**
3g **dietary fiber**
20g **protein**

- 1 teaspoon chili powder
- ½ teaspoon salt, divided
- 4 lean boneless pork chops (about 1¼ pounds), well trimmed
- 2 cups diced tomatoes
- 1 cup chopped green, red or yellow bell pepper
- ¾ cup thinly sliced celery
- ½ cup chopped onion
- 1 teaspoon dried thyme
- 1 tablespoon hot pepper sauce
- 2 tablespoons finely chopped fresh parsley

1. Rub chili powder and ¼ teaspoon salt evenly over one side of pork chops.

2. Combine tomatoes, bell peppers, celery, onion, thyme and hot pepper sauce in medium bowl; mix well.

3. Lightly spray large nonstick skillet with nonstick cooking spray; heat over medium-high heat. Add pork, seasoned side down; cook 1 minute. Turn pork. Top with tomato mixture; bring to a boil. Reduce heat to low. Cover; cook 25 minutes or until pork is tender and tomato mixture has thickened.

4. Transfer pork to serving plates. Bring tomato mixture to a boil over high heat; cook 2 minutes or until most liquid has evaporated. Remove from heat; stir in parsley and remaining ¼ teaspoon salt. Spoon sauce over pork.

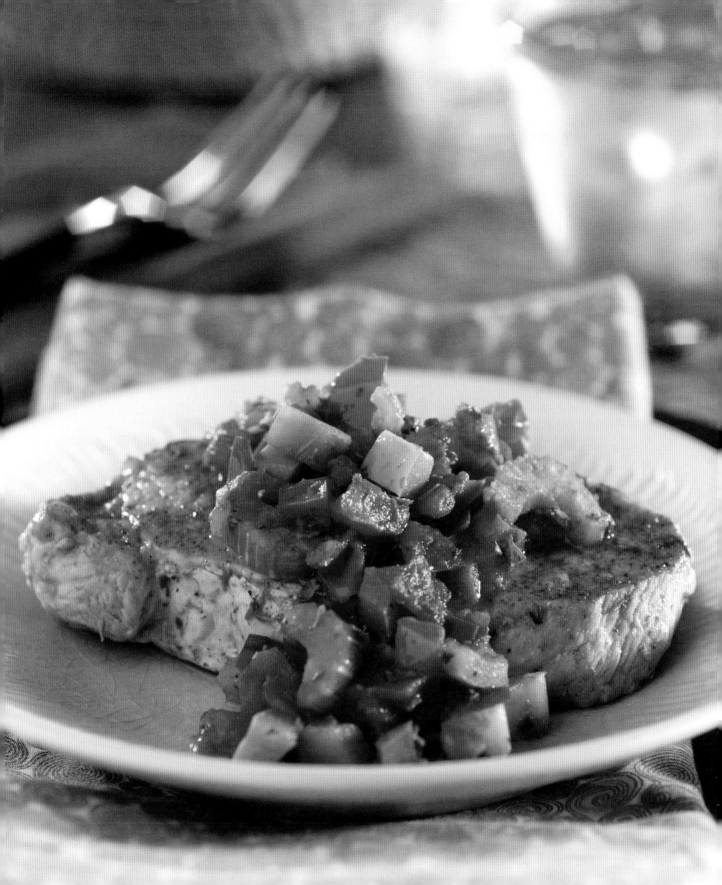

Stir-Fried Beef & Spinach

Makes 2 servings

PER SERVING

200 **calories**
5g **total fat**
14g **carbs**
12g **net carbs**
2g **dietary fiber**
27g **protein**

1 **package (6 ounces) fresh spinach, stemmed and torn**

8 **ounces boneless beef top sirloin steak, thinly sliced**

¼ **cup stir-fry sauce**

1 **teaspoon sugar**

½ **teaspoon curry powder**

¼ **teaspoon ground ginger**

1. Spray large skillet or wok with nonstick cooking spray; heat over high heat. Add spinach; stir-fry 1 minute or until wilted. Transfer spinach to serving platter. Keep warm.

2. Spray same skillet with cooking spray; heat over high heat. Add beef; stir-fry 2 minutes or until barely pink. Add stir-fry sauce, sugar, curry powder and ginger; cook and stir 1½ minutes or until sauce thickens. Serve with spinach.

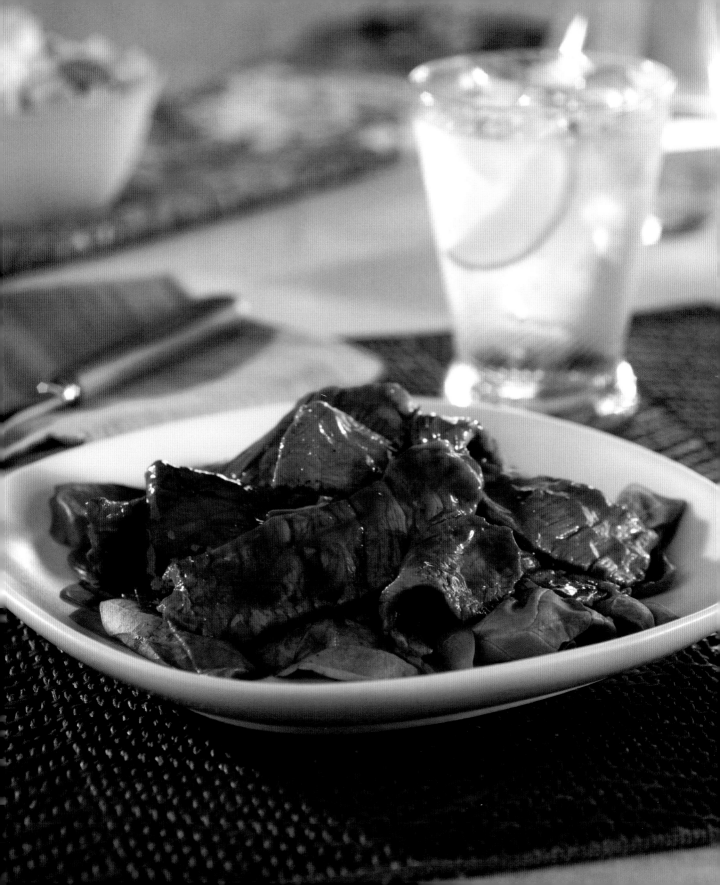

Greek-Style Beef Kabobs

Makes 4 servings

PER SERVING

193 **calories**
8g **total fat**
5g **carbs**
4g **net carbs**
1g **dietary fiber**
25g **protein**

 1 **pound boneless beef top sirloin steak (1 inch thick), cut into 16 pieces**

 ¼ **cup fat-free Italian salad dressing**

 3 **tablespoons fresh lemon juice, divided**

 1 **tablespoon dried oregano**

 1 **tablespoon Worcestershire sauce**

 2 **teaspoons dried basil**

 1 **teaspoon grated lemon peel**

 ⅛ **teaspoon red pepper flakes**

 1 **large green bell pepper, cut into 16 pieces**

16 **cherry tomatoes**

 2 **teaspoons olive oil**

 ⅛ **teaspoon salt**

1. Combine beef, salad dressing, 2 tablespoons lemon juice, oregano, Worcestershire sauce, basil, lemon peel and red pepper flakes in large resealable food storage bag. Seal bag; turn to coat. Marinate in refrigerator at least 8 hours or overnight, turning occasionally.

2. Preheat broiler. Remove beef from marinade; reserve marinade. Thread four 10-inch skewers with beef, alternating with bell pepper and tomatoes. Spray rimmed baking sheet or broiler pan with nonstick cooking spray. Brush kabobs with marinade; place on baking sheet. Discard remaining marinade. Broil kabobs 3 minutes. Turn over; broil 2 minutes or until desired doneness is reached. ***Do not overcook.*** Remove skewers to serving platter.

3. Add remaining 1 tablespoon lemon juice, oil and salt to pan drippings on baking sheet; stir well, scraping bottom of pan with flat spatula. Pour juices over kabobs.

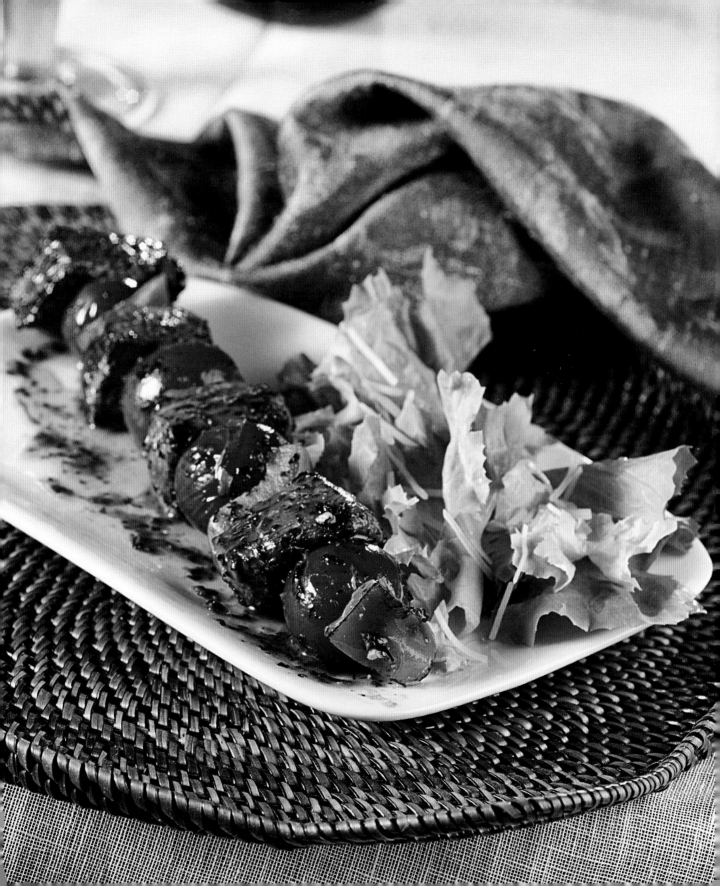

French Quarter Steaks

Makes 2 servings

- ½ cup water
- 2 tablespoons Worcestershire sauce
- 2 tablespoons soy sauce
- 1 tablespoon chili powder
- 3 cloves garlic, minced, divided
- 2 teaspoons paprika
- 1½ teaspoons ground red pepper
- 1¼ teaspoons black pepper, divided
- 1 teaspoon onion powder
- 2 top sirloin steaks (about 8 ounces each, 1 inch thick)
- 3 tablespoons butter, divided
- 1 tablespoon olive oil
- 1 large onion, thinly sliced
- 8 ounces sliced mushrooms (white and shiitake or all white)
- ¼ teaspoon plus ⅛ teaspoon salt, divided

1. Combine water, Worcestershire sauce, soy sauce, chili powder, 2 cloves garlic, paprika, red pepper, 1 teaspoon black pepper and onion powder in small bowl; mix well. Place steaks in large resealable food storage bag; pour marinade over steaks. Seal bag; turn to coat. Marinate in refrigerator 1 to 3 hours.

2. Remove steaks from marinade 30 minutes before cooking; discard marinade and pat steaks dry with paper towel. Prepare grill for direct cooking. Oil grid.

3. While grill is preheating, heat 1 tablespoon butter and oil in large skillet over medium high heat. Add onion; cook 5 minutes, stirring occasionally. Add mushrooms, ¼ teaspoon salt and remaining ¼ teaspoon black pepper; cook 10 minutes or until onion is golden brown and mushrooms are beginning to brown, stirring occasionally. Combine remaining 2 tablespoons butter, 1 clove garlic and ⅛ teaspoon salt in small skillet; cook over medium-low heat 3 minutes or until garlic begins to sizzle.

4. Grill steaks over medium-high heat 6 minutes; turn and cook 6 minutes for medium rare or until desired doneness. Brush both sides of steaks with garlic butter during last 2 minutes of cooking. Remove to plate and tent with foil; let rest 5 minutes. Serve steaks with onion and mushroom mixture.

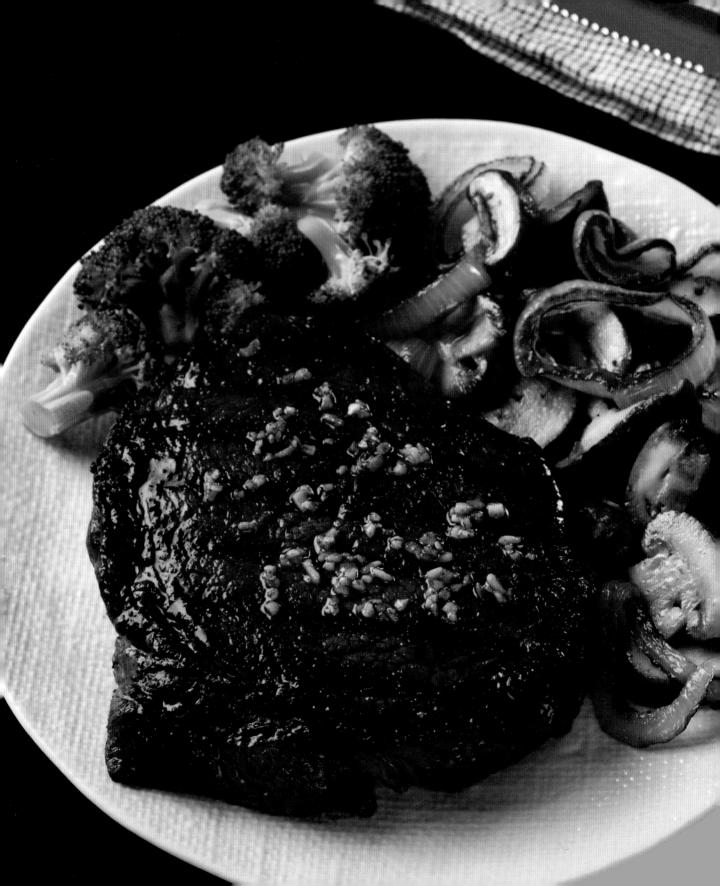

Bacon and Onion Brisket

Makes 6 servings

PER SERVING

360 **calories**
18g **total fat**
5g **carbs**
4g **net carbs**
1g **dietary fiber**
45g **protein**

6 slices bacon, cut crosswise into ½-inch strips

Salt and black pepper

1 flat-cut boneless beef brisket (about 2½ pounds)

3 medium onions, sliced

2 cans (about 14 ounces each) beef broth

Slow Cooker Directions

1. Cook bacon in large skillet over medium-high heat about 3 minutes. ***Do not overcook.*** Transfer bacon with slotted spoon to 5-quart slow cooker.

2. Season brisket with salt and pepper. Sear brisket in hot bacon fat on all sides, turning as it browns. Transfer to slow cooker.

3. Lower skillet heat to medium. Add onions to skillet. Cook and stir 3 to 5 minutes or until softened. Add to slow cooker. Pour in broth. Cover; cook on HIGH 6 to 8 hours or until meat is tender.

4. Transfer brisket to cutting board; let rest 10 minutes. Slice brisket against the grain into thin slices, and arrange on platter. Season with salt and pepper. Spoon bacon, onions and cooking liquid over brisket to serve.

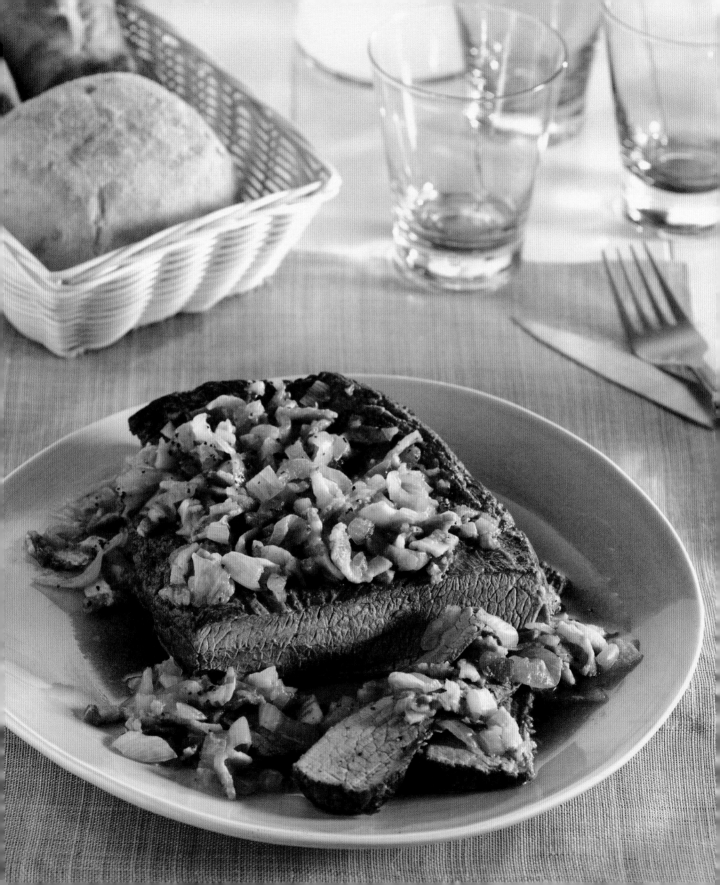

Herbed Lamb Chops

Makes 4 to 6 servings

⅓ cup olive oil

⅓ cup red wine vinegar

2 tablespoons soy sauce

1 tablespoon lemon juice

3 cloves garlic, crushed

1 teaspoon salt

1 teaspoon chopped fresh oregano *or* ¼ teaspoon dried oregano

1 teaspoon dried rosemary

1 teaspoon ground mustard

½ teaspoon white pepper

8 lamb loin chops, 1 inch thick (about 2 pounds)

1. Combine all ingredients except lamb in large resealable food storage bag. Reserve ½ cup marinade in small bowl. Add lamb to remaining marinade. Seal bag; turn to coat. Marinate in refrigerator at least 1 hour.

2. Prepare grill for direct cooking over medium-high heat.

3. Remove lamb from marinade; discard marinade. Grill lamb over medium-high heat 8 minutes or to desired doneness, turning once and basting often with reserved ½ cup marinade. *Do not baste during last 5 minutes of cooking.* Discard any remaining marinade.

Serving Suggestion: Serve with mashed cauliflower and a fresh green vegetable.

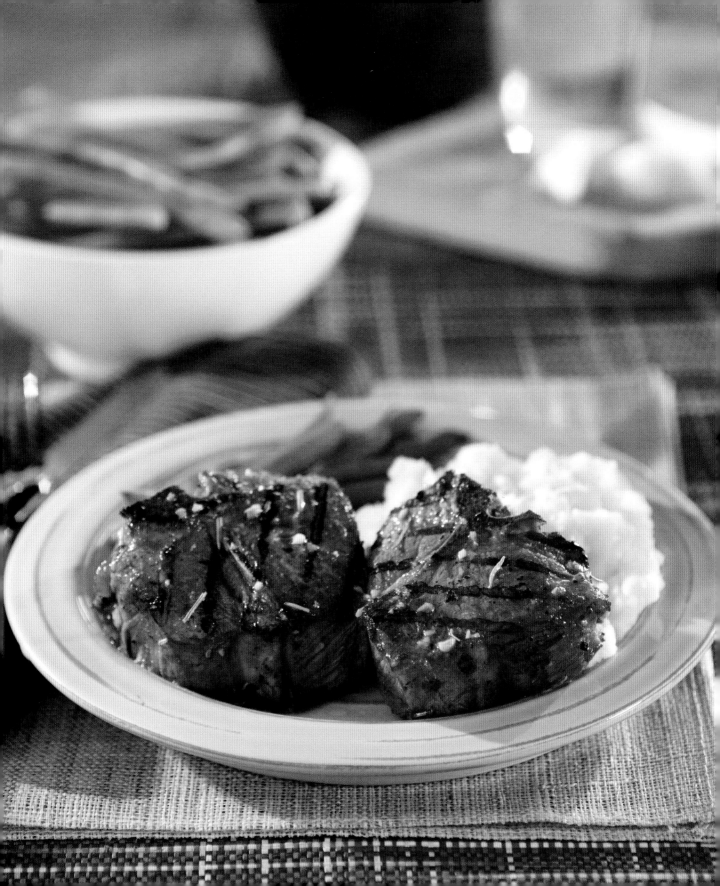

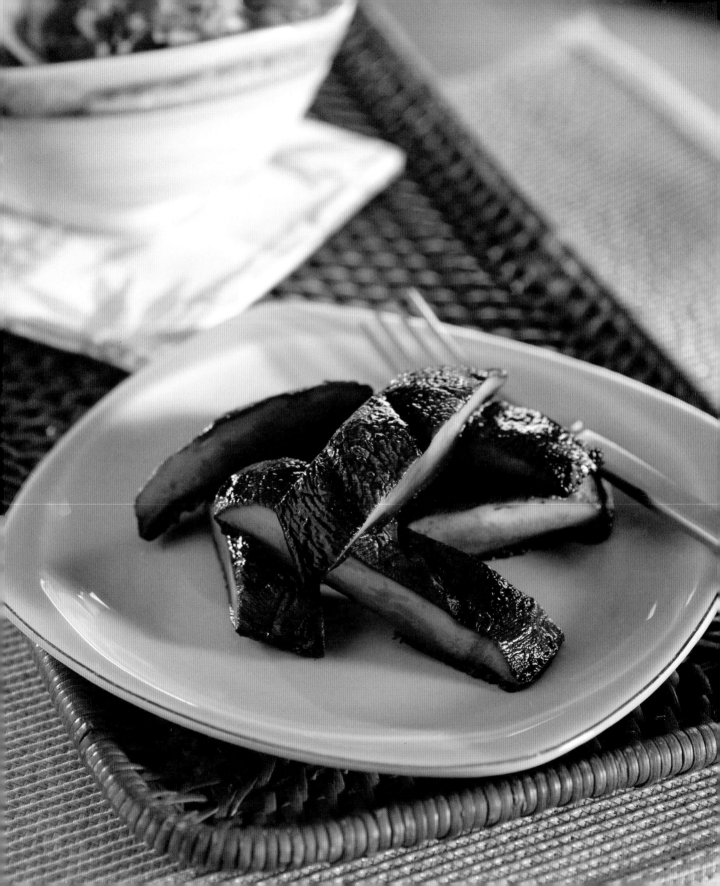

side dishes

PER SERVING

67 calories
2g total fat
9g carbs
8g net carbs
1g dietary fiber
4g protein

Portobello Mushrooms Sesame

Makes 4 servings

- 4 large portobello mushrooms
- 2 tablespoons sweet rice wine
- 2 tablespoons reduced-sodium soy sauce
- 2 cloves garlic, minced
- 1 teaspoon dark sesame oil

1. Prepare grill for direct cooking over medium heat.

2. Remove and discard stems from mushrooms; set caps aside. Whisk wine, soy sauce, garlic and oil in small bowl until well blended.

3. Brush both sides of mushroom caps with soy sauce mixture. Cook, top sides up, covered, 3 to 4 minutes. Brush tops with soy sauce mixture; turn and cook 2 minutes or until grill marks appear. Turn again and cook 4 to 5 minutes or until tender, basting frequently. Remove mushrooms; cut diagonally into ½-inch-thick slices.

Asparagus with Red Onion, Basil and Almonds

Makes 4 servings

PER SERVING

60 calories
4g total fat
6g carbs
4g net carbs
2g dietary fiber
3g protein

- 2 teaspoons butter
- ½ cup thinly sliced red onion, separated into rings
- 1 pound fresh asparagus, trimmed and cut into 1½-inch pieces
- ¼ cup reduced-sodium chicken broth
- 2 tablespoons chopped fresh basil
- ¼ teaspoon salt (optional)
- ¼ teaspoon black pepper
- 2 tablespoons sliced almonds, toasted*

*To toast almonds, place in nonstick skillet. Cook and stir over medium-low heat until nuts begin to brown, about 5 minutes. Remove immediately to plate to cool.

1. Melt butter in medium skillet over medium heat. Add onions. Cover; cook 5 minutes or until wilted. Uncover; cook 4 to 5 minutes, stirring occasionally, until onion is tender and golden brown.

2. Place asparagus and broth in medium saucepan. Cover; bring to a boil over high heat. Reduce heat; simmer 4 minutes. Uncover; stir in onion. Cook about 2 minutes or until asparagus is crisp-tender and most liquid has evaporated. Stir in basil, salt, if desired, and pepper. Transfer to serving plate. Sprinkle with almonds.

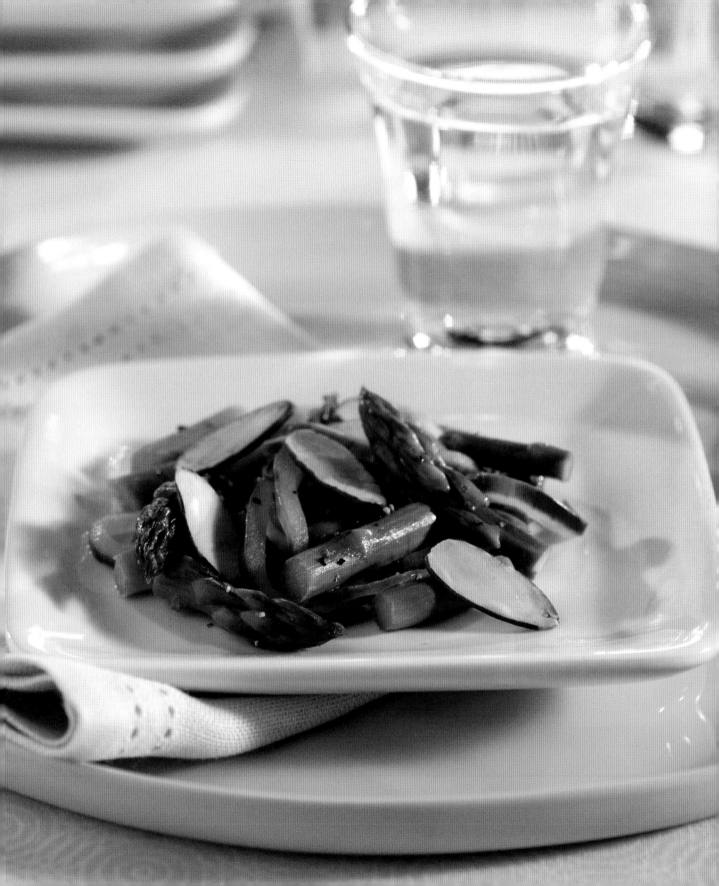

Collard Greens

Makes 10 servings

- **4** bunches collard greens, stemmed, washed and torn into bite-size pieces
- **2** cups water
- **½** medium red bell pepper, cut into strips
- **⅓** medium green bell pepper, cut into strips
- **¼** cup olive oil
- **¼** teaspoon salt
- **¼** teaspoon black pepper

Slow Cooker Directions

Combine all ingredients in slow cooker. Cover; cook on LOW 3 to 4 hours or on HIGH 2 hours or until done.

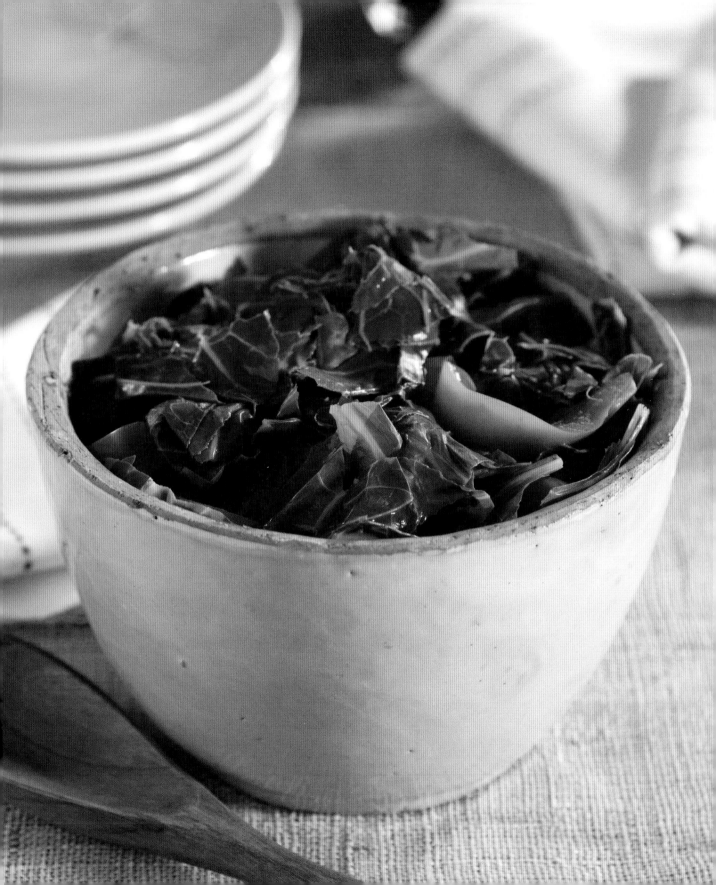

Barley & Vegetable Risotto

Makes 6 servings

PER SERVING

70 calories
3g **total fat**
7g **carbs**
5g **net carbs**
2g **dietary fiber**
3g **protein**

2 teaspoons olive oil

1 small onion, diced

8 ounces sliced mushrooms

¾ cup uncooked pearl barley

1 large red bell pepper, diced

4½ cups fat-free reduced-sodium vegetable or chicken broth

2 cups packed baby spinach

¼ cup grated Parmesan cheese

¼ teaspoon black pepper

Slow Cooker Directions

1. Heat oil in large nonstick skillet over medium-high heat. Add onion, cook and stir about 5 minutes or until lightly browned. Add mushrooms; cook 5 minutes, stirring frequently, or until mushrooms begin to brown. Transfer to slow cooker.

2. Add barley, bell pepper and broth. Cover; cook on LOW 4 to 5 hours or on HIGH 2½ to 3 hours or until barley is tender and liquid is absorbed. Stir in spinach. Let stand 5 minutes. Gently stir in Parmesan cheese and black pepper just before serving.

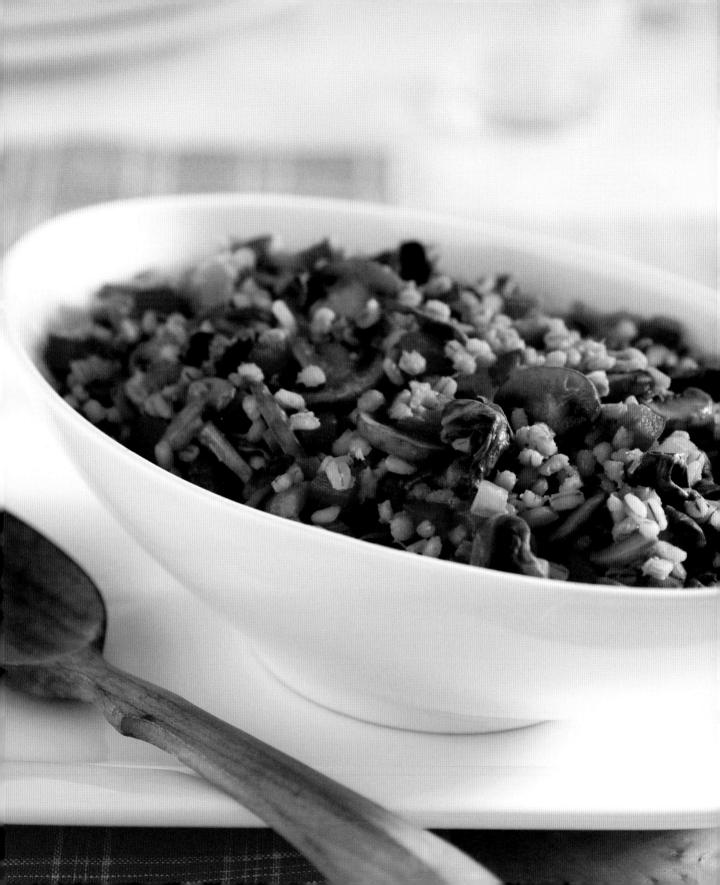

Great Zukes Pizza Bites

Makes 8 servings (2 bites per serving)

1 **medium zucchini**

3 **tablespoons pizza sauce**

2 **tablespoons tomato paste**

¼ **teaspoon dried oregano**

¾ **cup (3 ounces) shredded mozzarella cheese**

¼ **cup shredded Parmesan cheese**

8 **slices pitted black olives**

8 **slices pepperoni**

1. Preheat broiler; set rack 4 inches from heat.

2. Trim and discard ends of zucchini. Cut zucchini into 16 (¼-inch-thick) diagonal slices. Place on nonstick baking sheet.

3. Combine pizza sauce, tomato paste and oregano in small bowl; mix well. Spread scant teaspoon sauce over each zucchini slice. Combine cheeses in small bowl. Top each zucchini slice with 1 tablespoon cheese mixture, pressing down into sauce. Place 1 olive slice on each of eight pizza bites. Place 1 folded pepperoni slice on each remaining pizza bite.

4. Broil 3 minutes or until cheese is melted. Serve immediately.

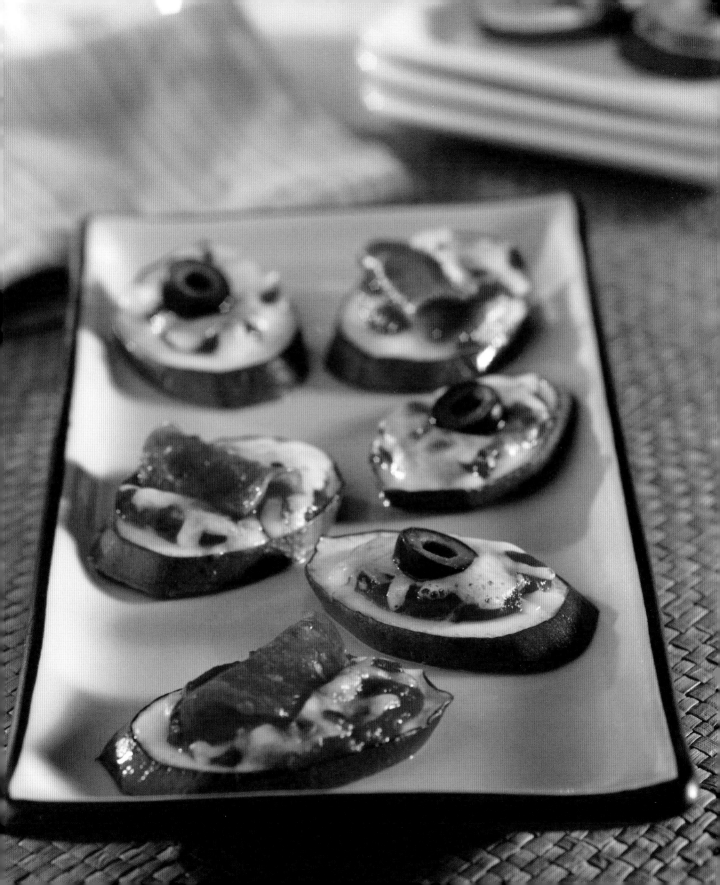

Beet Chips

Makes 3 servings

PER SERVING

100 **calories**
7g **total fat**
8g **carbs**
6g **net carbs**
2g **dietary fiber**
1g **protein**

3 **medium beets (red and/or golden), trimmed**

1½ **tablespoons extra virgin olive oil**

¼ **teaspoon salt**

¼ **teaspoon black pepper**

1. Preheat oven to 300°F.

2. Cut beets into very thin slices, about ¹⁄₁₆ inch thick. Combine beets, oil, salt and pepper in medium bowl; gently toss to coat. Arrange in single layer on baking sheet.

3. Bake 30 to 35 minutes or until darkened and crisp.* Spread on paper towels to cool completely.

*If the beet chips are darkened but not crisp, turn oven off and let chips stand in oven until crisp, about 10 minutes. Do not keep the oven on as the chips will burn easily.

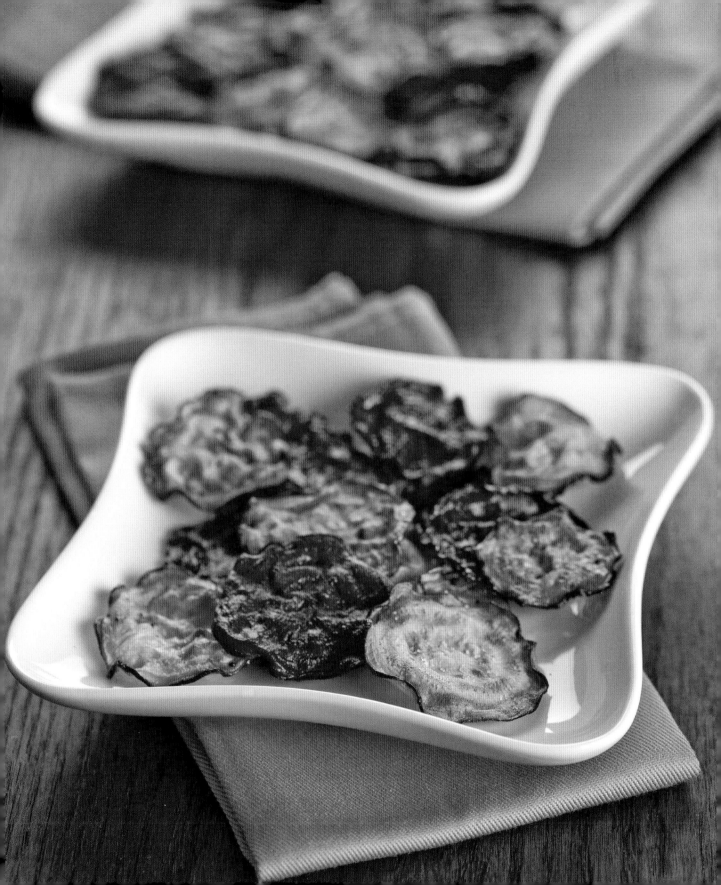

Tofu Cauliflower Fried Rice

Makes 4 servings

- 3 **tablespoons soy sauce**
- 1 **tablespoon plus 1 teaspoon minced fresh ginger, divided**
- 2 **teaspoons dark sesame oil**
- 1 **teaspoon packed brown sugar**
- 1 **teaspoon rice vinegar**
- 1 **package (14 ounces) firm tofu, drained and cut into 1-inch cubes**
- 2 **tablespoons vegetable oil, divided**
- 1 **yellow or sweet onion, chopped**
- 1 **carrot, chopped**
- ½ **cup frozen peas**
- 2 **cloves garlic, minced**
- 1 **package (12 ounces) frozen cauliflower rice**
- 1 **green onion, thinly sliced**

1. Whisk soy sauce, 1 tablespoon ginger, sesame oil, brown sugar and vinegar in small bowl. Place tofu in quart-size resealable food storage bag. Pour marinade over tofu. Seal bag, pressing out as much air as possible. Turn to coat tofu with marinade. Refrigerate 3 hours or overnight.

2. Drain tofu, reserving marinade. Heat 1 tablespoon vegetable oil in large skillet over high heat. Add tofu; stir-fry 3 to 5 minutes or until edges are browned. Transfer to bowl.

3. Heat remaining 1 tablespoon vegetable oil in same skillet. Add onion and carrot; stir-fry 2 minutes or until softened. Add peas, garlic and remaining 1 teaspoon ginger; cook 2 minutes or until peas are hot. Add cauliflower rice and ¼ cup reserved marinade; stir-fry 5 minutes or until heated through. Return tofu to skillet; stir-fry until heated through. Top with green onion.

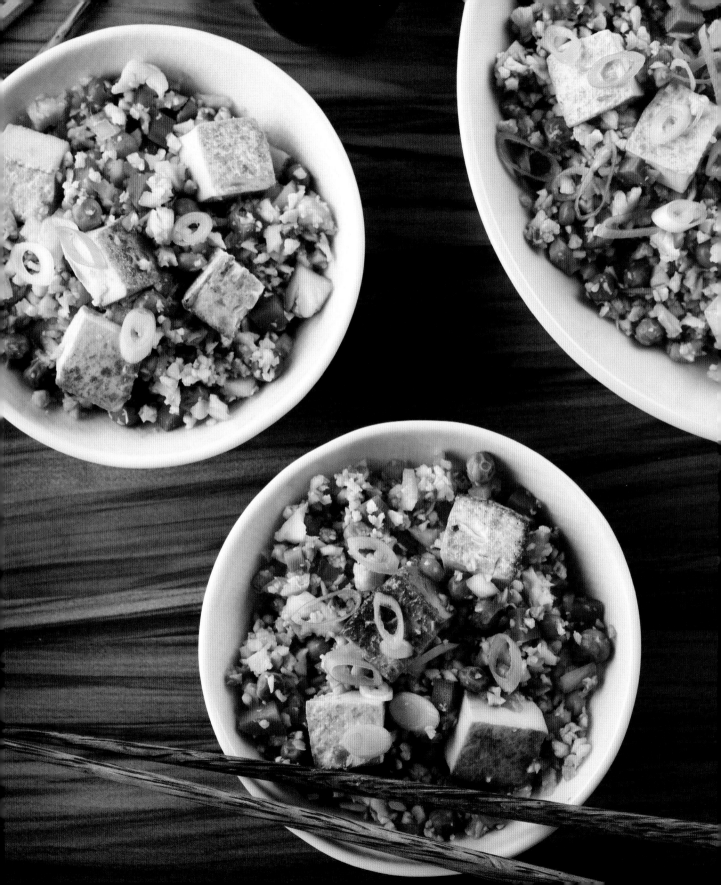

Brussels Sprouts with Bacon and Butter

Makes 4 servings

PER SERVING

220 **calories**
15g **total fat**
15g **carbs**
8g **net carbs**
7g **dietary fiber**
10g **protein**

6 slices thick-cut bacon, cut into ½-inch pieces

1½ pounds Brussels sprouts (about 24 medium), halved

¼ teaspoon salt

¼ teaspoon black pepper

2 tablespoons butter, softened

1. Preheat oven to 375°F. Cook bacon in large cast iron skillet until almost crisp. Drain on paper towel-lined plate; set aside. Drain all but 1 tablespoon drippings.

2. Add Brussels sprouts to skillet. Sprinkle with salt and pepper; toss to coat. Spread in skillet.

3. Roast 30 minutes or until Brussels sprouts are browned and crispy, stirring every 10 minutes.

4. Add butter to skillet; stir until completely coated. Stir in bacon.

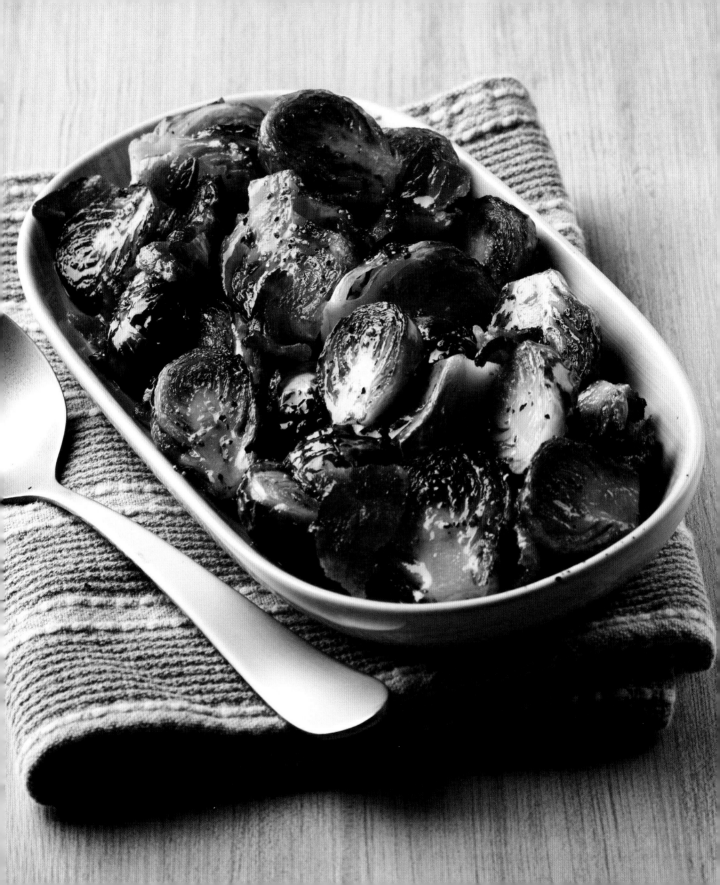

Zoodles in Tomato Sauce

Makes 8 servings

PER SERVING

70 **calories**
3g **total fat**
8g **carbs**
5g **net carbs**
3g **dietary fiber**
4g **protein**

3 teaspoons olive oil, divided

2 cloves garlic

1 tablespoon tomato paste

1 can (28 ounces) whole tomatoes, undrained

1 teaspoon dried oregano

½ teaspoon salt

2 large zucchini (about 16 ounces each), ends trimmed, cut into 3-inch pieces

¼ cup shredded Parmesan cheese

1. Heat 2 teaspoons oil in medium saucepan over medium heat. Add garlic; cook 1 minute or until fragrant but not browned. Stir in tomato paste; cook 30 seconds, stirring constantly. Add tomatoes with juice, oregano and salt; break up tomatoes with wooden spoon. Bring to a simmer. Reduce heat; cook 30 minutes or until thickened.

2. Meanwhile, spiral zucchini with fine spiral blade.* Heat remaining 1 teaspoon oil in large skillet over medium-high heat. Add zucchini; cook 4 to 5 minutes or until tender, stirring frequently. Transfer to serving plates; top with tomato sauce and Parmesan cheese.

*If you don't have a spiralizer, cut the zucchini into ribbons with a mandoline or sharp knife. Or for small wedges that mimic a small pasta shape, cut it lengthwise into quarters and then thinly slice it crosswise.

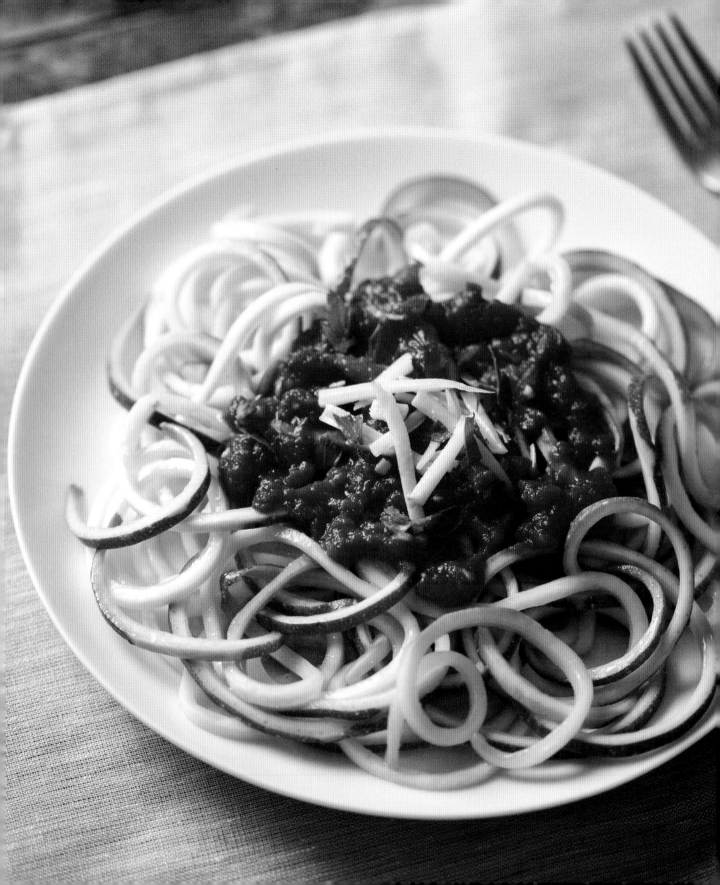

Savory Zucchini Sticks

Makes 4 servings

- 6 **tablespoons almond flour**
- ¼ **cup grated Parmesan cheese**
- 1 **egg white**
- 1 **tablespoon water**
- 2 **small zucchini (about 4 ounces each), cut lengthwise into quarters**
- ⅓ **cup pasta sauce, warmed**

1. Preheat oven to 400°F. Spray baking sheet with nonstick cooking spray.

2. Combine almond flour and Parmesan cheese in shallow dish. Combine egg white and water in another shallow dish; beat with fork until well blended.

3. Dip each piece of zucchini into egg white mixture, letting excess drip back into dish. Roll in crumb mixture to coat. Place zucchini sticks on prepared baking sheet; spray with cooking spray.

4. Bake 15 to 18 minutes or until golden brown. Serve with pasta sauce.

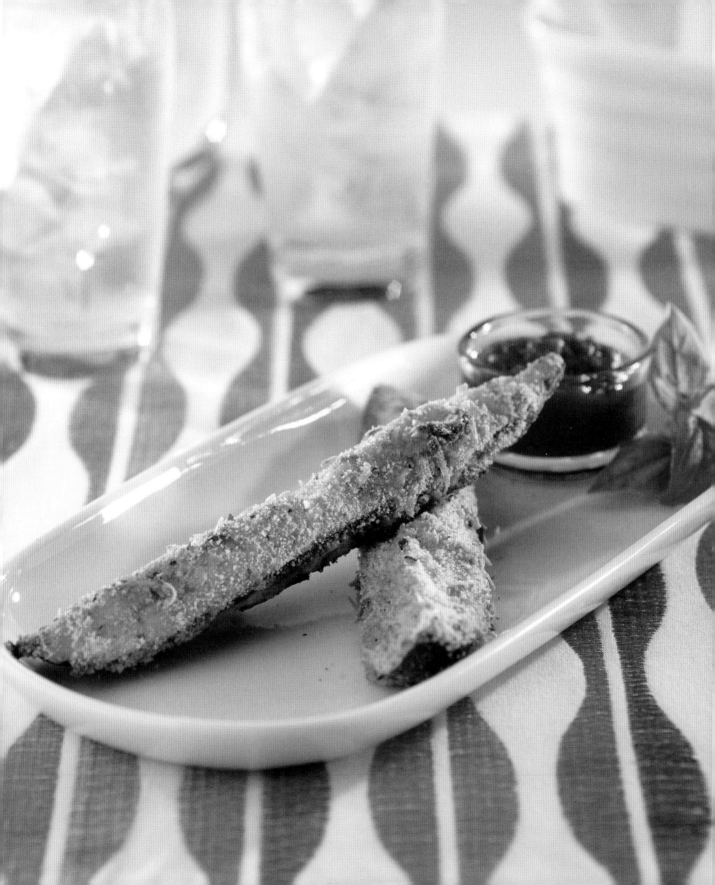

Twice Baked Loaded Cauliflower

Makes 8 servings

PER SERVING

250 calories
18g total fat
12g carbs
7g net carbs
5g dietary fiber
13g protein

2 heads cauliflower, cut into florets (8 cups)

2 tablespoons vegetable or olive oil

1 teaspoon salt

¼ cup (½ stick) butter, cut into small pieces

¼ cup milk

½ cup chopped green onions, divided

1 cup (4 ounces) shredded Cheddar cheese, divided

4 ounces bacon, crisp cooked and crumbled

½ cup chopped tomatoes

Sour cream

1. Preheat oven to 425°F. Divide cauliflower between two 13×9-inch baking pans. Drizzle each with 1 tablespoon oil and sprinkle each with ½ teaspoon salt. Roast 40 minutes, stirring cauliflower and rotating pans once. ***Reduce oven temperature to 375°F.***

2. Transfer cauliflower to food processor; add butter and milk. Process 1 to 2 minutes or until very smooth and fluffy. Stir in half of green onions and ½ cup cheese. Divide mixture among eight ramekins. Sprinkle with remaining cheese and bacon. Bake 10 to 15 minutes or until cheese is melted and browned around edge and cauliflower is heated through. Top with remaining green onions, tomatoes and sour cream.

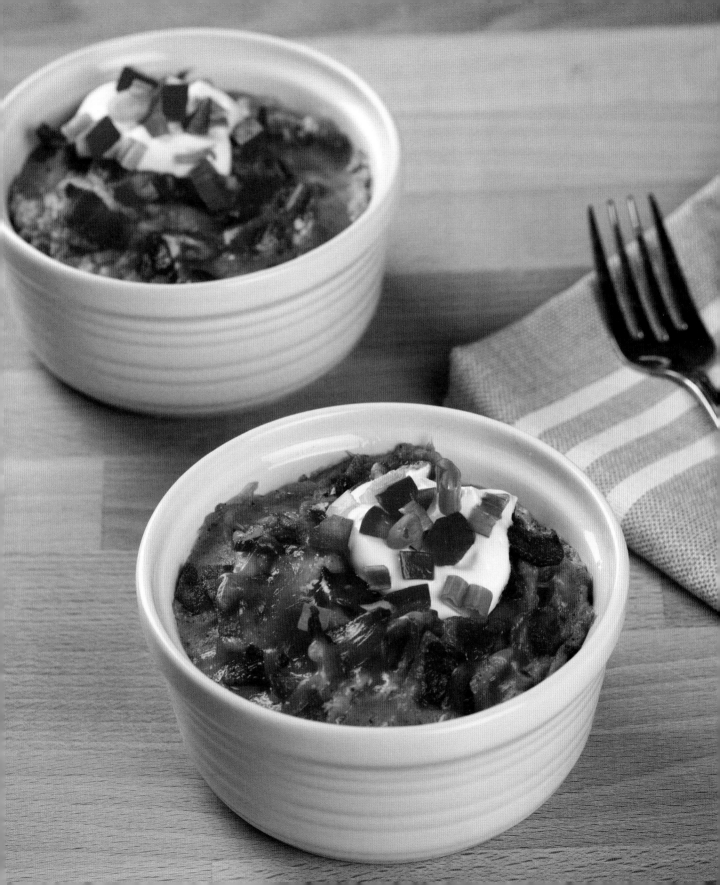

Garlic "Bread" Sticks

Makes 14 servings

PER SERVING

110 **calories**
8g **total fat**
4g **carbs**
3g **net carbs**
1g **dietary fiber**
8g **protein**

1 **medium head cauliflower, finely chopped and squeezed dry**

1 **cup (4 ounces) shredded mozzarella cheese**

1 **cup shredded Parmesan cheese, divided**

¾ **cup almond flour**

2 **cloves garlic, minced**

½ **teaspoon Italian seasoning**

1 **teaspoon salt**

1 **egg**

1. Preheat oven to 425°F. Line sheet pan with parchment paper or grease with 1 tablespoon vegetable oil.

2. Combine cauliflower, mozzarella, ½ cup Parmesan cheese, almond flour, garlic, Italian seasoning, salt and egg in large bowl; mix well. Pat into 12×10-inch rectangle on prepared sheet pan.

3. Bake 30 minutes or until well browned and edges are crispy. Sprinkle with additional ½ cup shredded Parmesan. Bake 10 minutes or until cheese is melted.

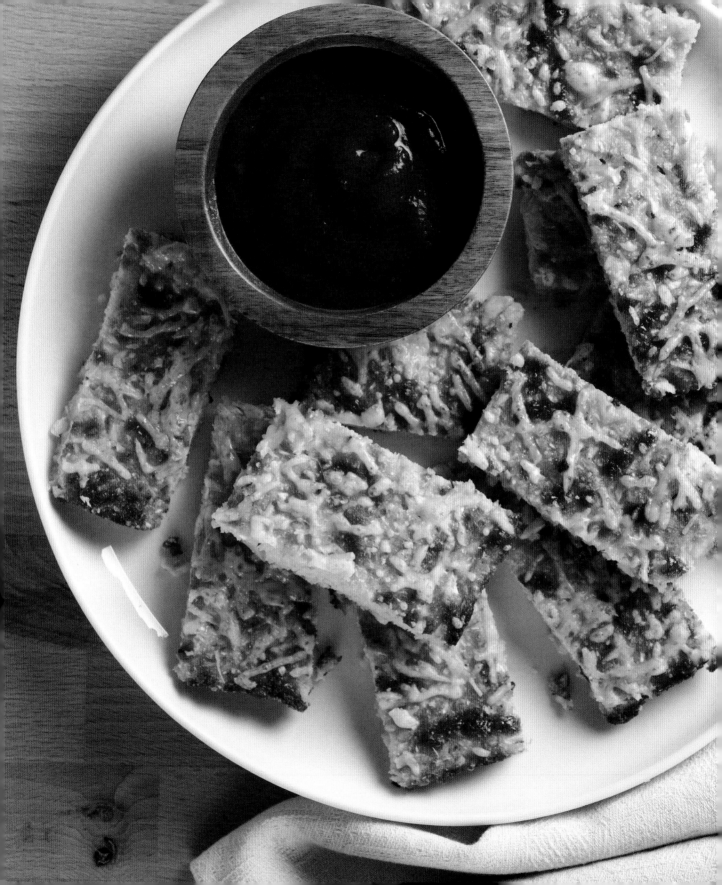

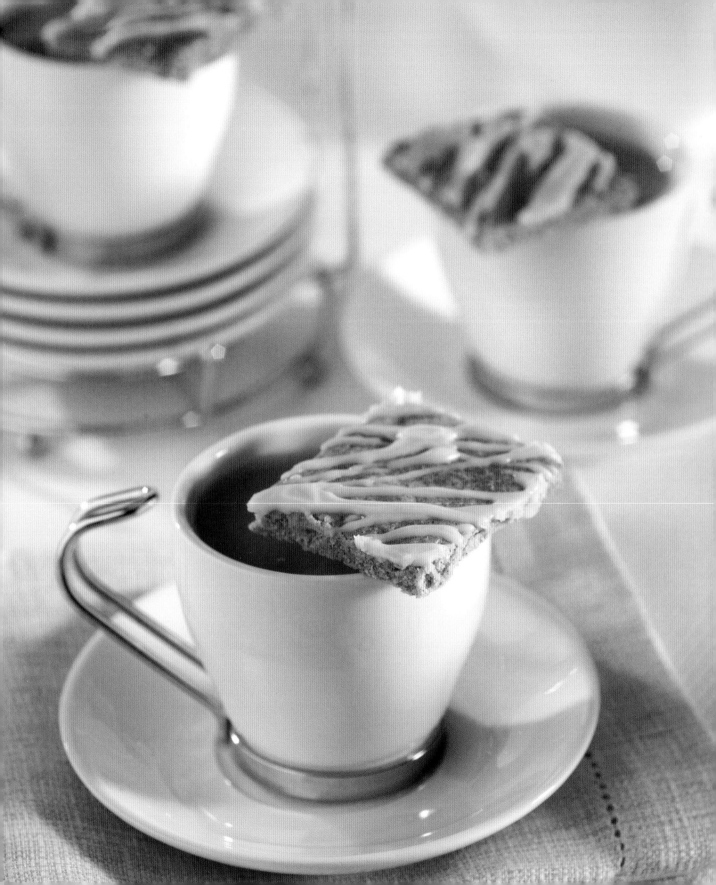

desserts

PER SERVING

60 calories
2g **total fat**
9g **carbs**
9g **net carbs**
0g **dietary fiber**
1g **protein**

Cinnamon Flats

Makes 50 cookies (1 per serving)

1¾ **cups all-purpose flour**

½ **cup granulated sugar**

1½ **teaspoons ground cinnamon**

¼ **teaspoon salt**

¼ **teaspoon ground nutmeg**

½ **cup (1 stick) cold margarine**

3 **egg whites, divided**

1 **teaspoon vanilla**

1 **teaspoon water**

Sugar Glaze (recipe follows)

1. Preheat oven to 350°F. Spray 15×10-inch jelly roll pan with nonstick cooking spray. Combine flour, granulated sugar, cinnamon, salt and nutmeg in medium bowl. Cut in margarine with pastry blender or two knives until mixture forms coarse crumbs. Beat in 2 egg whites and vanilla; mix to form soft dough.

2. Divide dough into six equal pieces; place on prepared pan. Press dough evenly to edges of pan; smooth top of dough with metal spatula. Mix remaining egg white and water in small cup; brush over dough. Lightly score dough into 2×1½-inch pieces.

3. Prepare Sugar Glaze. Bake 20 to 25 minutes or until lightly browned and firm. While still warm, cut along score lines into pieces; drizzle with Sugar Glaze. Let stand 15 minutes or until glaze is firm before removing from pan.

Sugar Glaze: Combine ½ cups powdered sugar, 2 tablespoons fat-free (skim) milk and 1 teaspoon vanilla in small bowl. If glaze is too thick, add additional 1 tablespoon milk.

Fruit Freezies

Makes 12 servings (2 per serving)

PER SERVING

19 calories
1g total fat
5g carbs
4g net carbs
1g dietary fiber
1g protein

1   can (15 ounces) apricot halves in light syrup, rinsed and drained

¾   cup apricot nectar

3   tablespoons sugar, divided
    Ice cube trays (round or square)

1   can (15 ounces) sliced pears in light syrup, rinsed and drained

¾   cup pear nectar

1½   cups frozen chopped mango

¾   cup mango nectar
    Picks or mini pop sticks

1. Combine apricots, apricot nectar and 1 tablespoon sugar in blender or food processor; blend until smooth. Pour mixture evenly into one third of ice cube trays.

2. Combine pears, pear nectar and 1 tablespoon sugar in blender or food processor; blend until smooth. Pour mixture evenly into one third of ice cube trays.

3. Combine mango, mango nectar and remaining 1 tablespoon sugar in blender or food processor; blend until smooth. Pour mixture evenly into remaining one third of ice cube trays.

4. Freeze 1 to 2 hours or until almost firm.

5. Insert picks. Freeze 1 to 2 hours or until firm.

6. To remove pops from trays, place bottoms of ice cube trays under warm running water until loosened. Press firmly on bottoms to release. (Do not twist or pull picks.)

Variation: Try any of these favorite fruit combinations or create your own! Use crushed pineapple and pineapple juice or add more flavor to the combinations above. Add coconut extract to the apricot mixture or almond extract to the pear mixture.

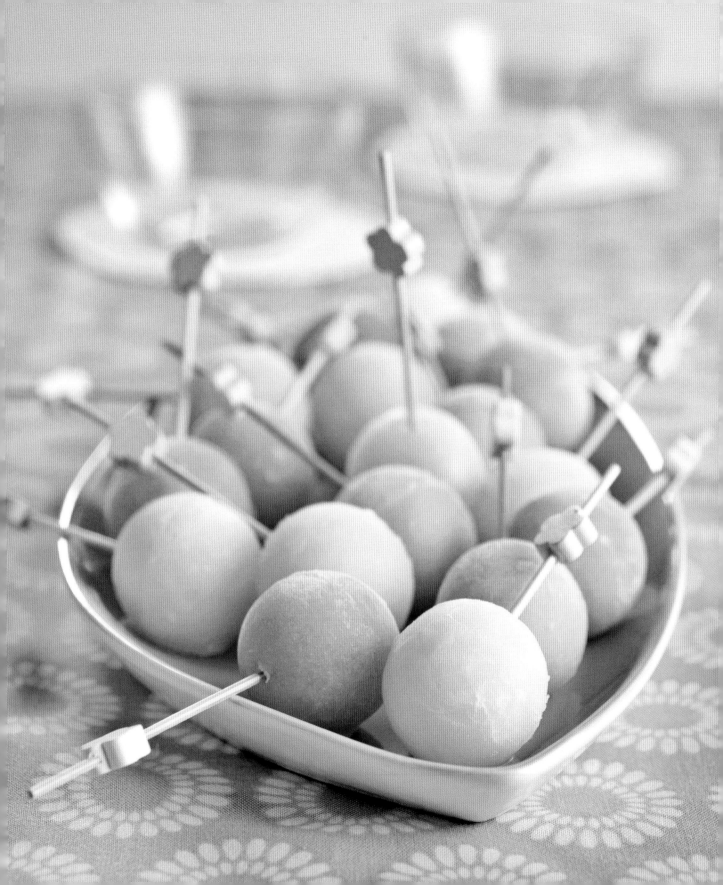

Cocoa Meringue Kisses

Makes 9 dozen cookies (3 cookies per serving)

½ cup raw hazelnuts

1 cup sugar, divided

5 tablespoons cocoa powder

3 tablespoons cornstarch

½ teaspoon ground cinnamon

¼ teaspoon grated nutmeg

3 egg whites, at room temperature

¼ teaspoon cream of tartar

1¼ teaspoons vanilla

3 ounces bittersweet chocolate, finely chopped

1. Preheat oven to 350°F. Place hazelnuts in cake or pie pan; bake 15 to 18 minutes or until skins split and nuts are golden. Transfer nuts to clean kitchen towel; rub nuts in towel to remove most of skins. Position racks in upper and lower thirds of oven. *Reduce oven temperature to 200°F.* Line two cookie sheets with foil.

2. Place hazelnuts and ⅓ cup sugar in food processor; process with on/off pulses about 2 minutes or until nuts are finely ground. Add cocoa, cornstarch, cinnamon and nutmeg; process with on/off pulses until blended.

3. Beat egg whites in clean bowl with electric mixer at medium-high speed until foamy. Add cream of tartar; beat until egg whites hold soft peaks. Gradually sprinkle with remaining ⅔ cup sugar; beat until egg whites hold firm and shiny, but not stiff, peaks. Stir in vanilla.

4. Fold hazelnut mixture into beaten egg whites in three parts, mixing well after each addition. Scoop 1-inch mounds onto prepared cookie sheets with spoon, leaving 1 inch between mounds.

5. Bake 45 minutes. Rotate cookie sheets top to bottom and front to back; bake 45 minutes. Turn oven off; leave meringues in oven 1 hour. Carefully peel meringues from foil and turn bottoms up.

6. Place chocolate in small microwavable bowl; microwave on LOW (30%) 30 seconds. Stir chocolate; microwave at additional 15-second intervals until melted, stirring frequently. Use pastry brush to coat bottoms of meringues with melted chocolate. Refrigerate 10 minutes to set chocolate. Warm remaining melted chocolate in microwave; brush bottom of meringues again with melted chocolate. Refrigerate 10 minutes to set. Store meringues tightly covered with foil up to 1 week.

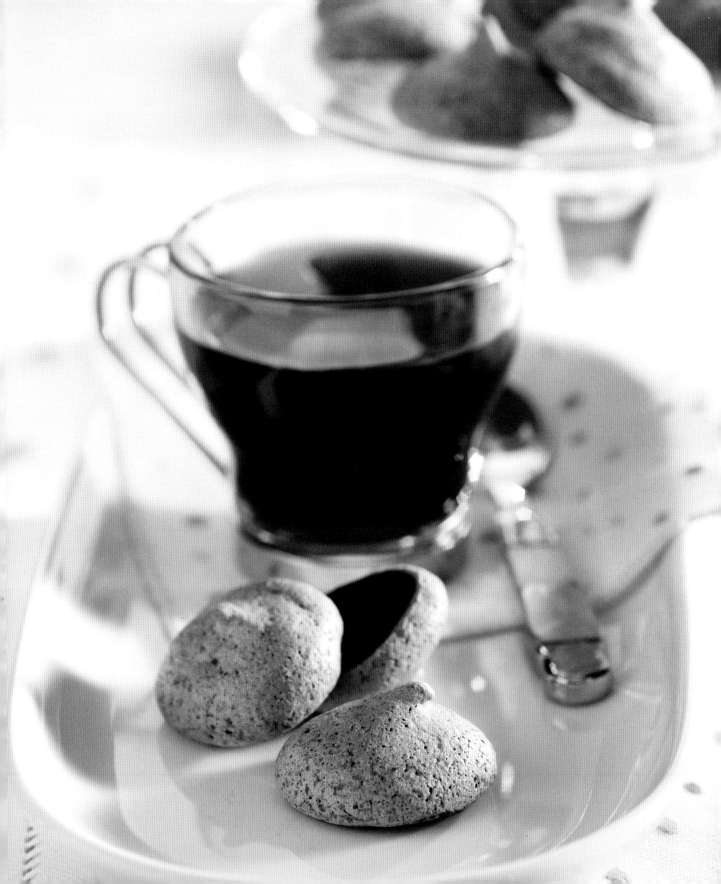

Lemon Soufflé Cake with Strawberry Sauce

Makes 6 servings

PER SERVING

212 **calories**
17g **total fat**
10g **carbs**
9g **net carbs**
1g **dietary fiber**
5g **protein**

½ cup ripe strawberries, diced and mashed

⅔ cup plus 2 teaspoons sugar substitute*

3 egg yolks, beaten

¼ cup strained fresh lemon juice

2 teaspoons grated lemon peel

¼ cup all-purpose flour

1 cup whipping cream

3 egg whites

½ teaspoon cream of tartar

6 sprigs fresh mint (optional)

*This recipe was tested with sucralose-based sugar substitute.

1. Preheat oven to 350°F. Spray six 8-ounce glass or ceramic ovenproof soufflé dishes with nonstick cooking spray.

2. Combine mashed strawberries and 2 teaspoons sugar substitute in small bowl. Stir until well mixed; set aside.

3. Combine egg yolks, remaining ⅔ cup sugar substitute, lemon juice, lemon peel and flour in medium bowl; beat until smooth. Stir in cream.

4. Combine egg whites and cream of tartar in clean bowl; beat with electric mixer at high speed until stiff peaks form. Gradually fold egg whites into lemon batter. Gently spoon (do not pour) batter evenly into prepared dishes.

5. Place dishes in 15×10×2-inch baking pan. Fill pan with hot water to halfway point on dishes. Bake 35 to 40 minutes or until tops are puffed, golden brown and spring back when touched lightly with finger. Remove from oven; let stand in baking pan 10 minutes.

6. Spoon 4 teaspoons strawberry sauce over each warm soufflé; garnish with mint.

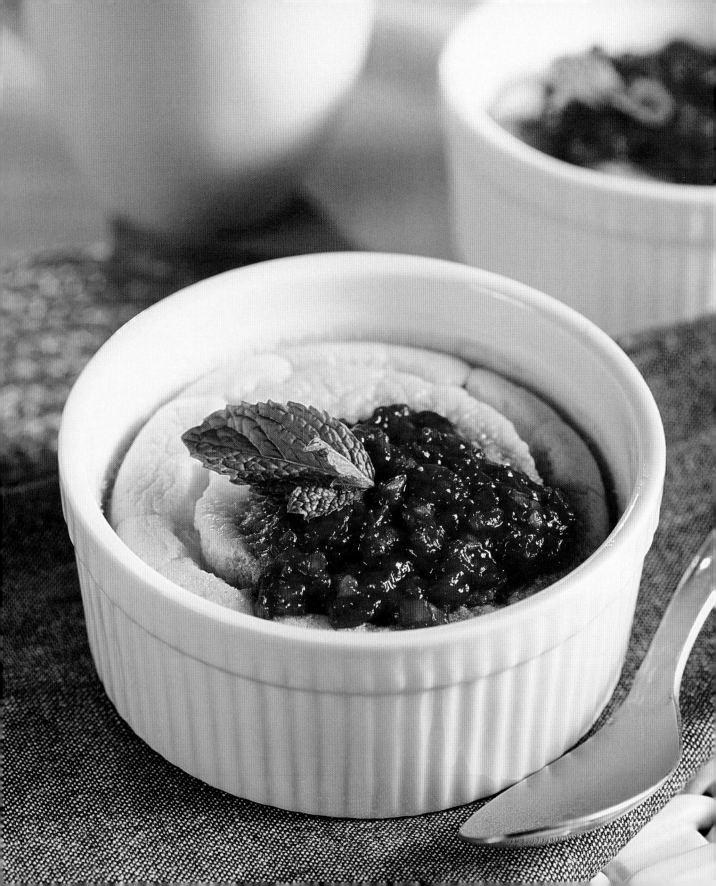

Chocolate-Almond Meringue Puffs

Makes 15 servings

- 2 tablespoons granulated sugar
- 3 packets sugar substitute*
- 1½ teaspoons unsweetened cocoa powder
- 2 egg whites, at room temperature
- ½ teaspoon vanilla
- ¼ teaspoon cream of tartar
- ¼ teaspoon almond extract
- ⅛ teaspoon salt
- 1½ ounces (7 tablespoons) sliced almonds
- 3 tablespoons seedless raspberry fruit spread

This recipe was tested with sucralose-based sugar substitute.

1. Preheat oven to 275°F. Line cookie sheet with foil. Combine granulated sugar, sugar substitute and cocoa in small bowl.

2. Beat egg whites in medium bowl with electric mixer at high speed until foamy. Add vanilla, cream of tartar, almond extract and salt; beat until soft peaks form. Add sugar mixture, 1 tablespoon at a time, beating until stiff peaks form.

3. Spoon 15 equal mounds of egg white mixture onto prepared cookie sheet. Sprinkle with almonds.

4. Bake 1 hour. Turn oven off but do not open door. Leave puffs in oven 2 hours longer or until completely dry. Remove from oven; cool completely.

5. Stir fruit spread; spoon about ½ teaspoon spread onto each meringue just before serving.

Tip: Puffs are best if eaten the same day they're made. If necessary, store in airtight container, adding fruit topping at time of serving.

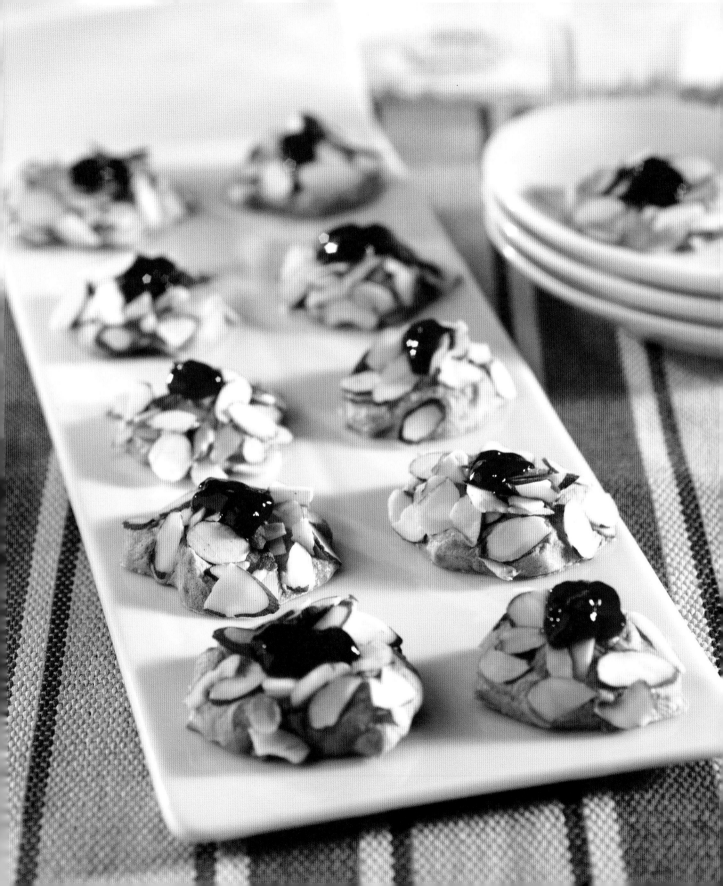

Coffee Granita

Makes 5 servings

PER SERVING

42 calories
1g total fat
8g carbs
8g net carbs
0g dietary fiber
1g protein

2 cups water

1½ tablespoons instant coffee

¼ cup powdered sugar

2 tablespoons sugar substitute*

5 tablespoons frozen thawed whipped topping or fat-free topping

This recipe was tested with sucralose-based sugar substitute.

1. Combine water, coffee, powdered sugar and sugar substitute in small saucepan. Bring to a boil over medium-high heat and stir to dissolve completely.

2. Pour into metal 8-inch square pan. Cover pan with foil and place in freezer. Freeze granita 2 hours or until slushy. Remove from freezer; stir to break mixture up into small chunks. Cover and return to freezer. Freeze 2 hours then stir to break granita up again. Cover and freeze at least 4 hours or overnight.

3. To serve, scrape surface of granita with large metal spoon to shave off thin pieces. Spoon into individual bowls. Top each serving with 1 tablespoon whipped topping. Serve immediately.

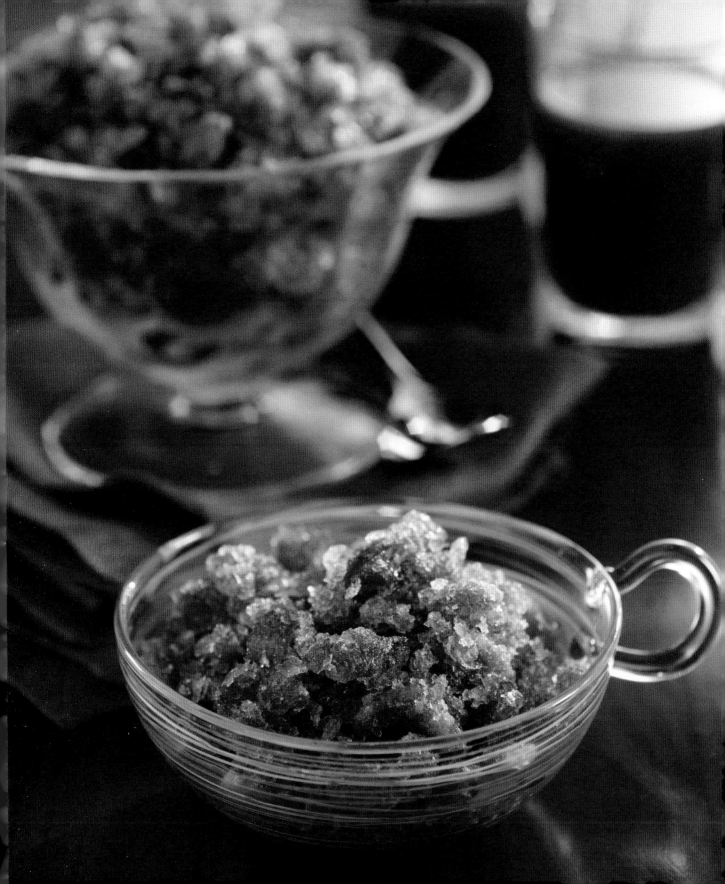

Blackberry Macaroons

Makes 4 dozen macaroons

PER SERVING

47 calories
3g **total fat**
5g **carbs**
4g **net carbs**
1g **dietary fiber**
2g **protein**

- 1 **package (14 ounces) sweetened flaked coconut**
- ¼ **cup all-purpose flour**
- ¼ **cup sugar**
- 2 **egg whites**
- ½ **teaspoon almond extract**
- 1 **cup fresh or frozen blackberries**

1. Preheat oven to 325°F. Line baking sheets with parchment paper.

2. Combine coconut, flour, sugar, egg whites and almond extract in food processor or blender; process until combined. Remove to medium bowl.

3. Gently mash blackberries in small bowl. (Some chunks may remain). Fold blackberries into coconut mixture just until combined. ***Do not overmix***.

4. Shape mixture into ½-inch balls. Place on prepared baking sheets.

5. Bake 25 to 27 minutes or until set. Remove to wire racks; cool completely.

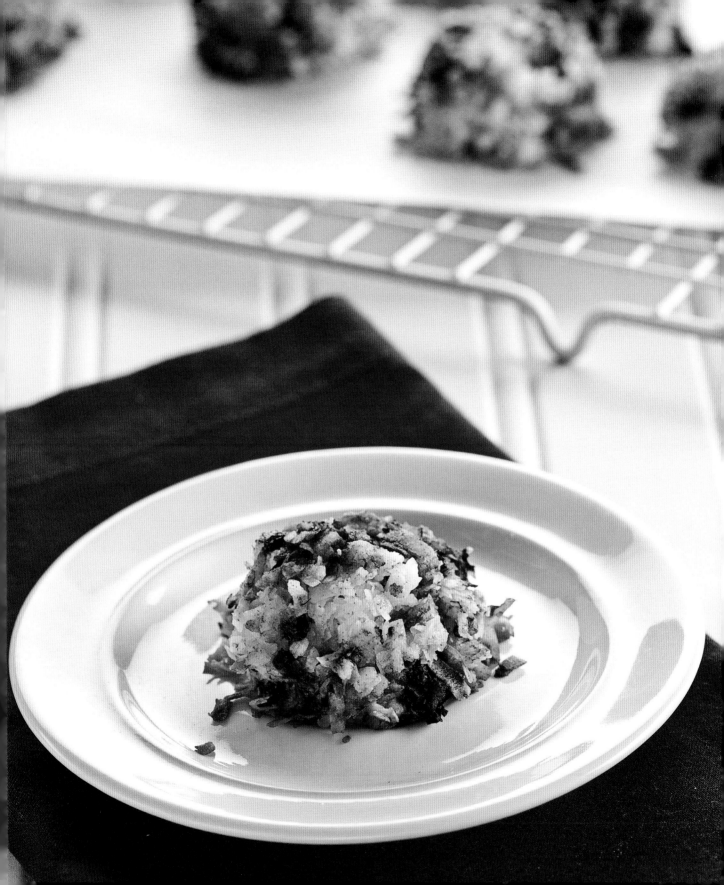

metric conversion chart

VOLUME MEASUREMENTS (dry)

1/8 teaspoon = 0.5 mL
1/4 teaspoon = 1 mL
1/2 teaspoon = 2 mL
3/4 teaspoon = 4 mL
1 teaspoon = 5 mL
1 tablespoon = 15 mL
2 tablespoons = 30 mL
1/4 cup = 60 mL
1/3 cup = 75 mL
1/2 cup = 125 mL
2/3 cup = 150 mL
3/4 cup = 175 mL
1 cup = 250 mL
2 cups = 1 pint = 500 mL
3 cups = 750 mL
4 cups = 1 quart = 1 L

VOLUME MEASUREMENTS (fluid)

1 fluid ounce (2 tablespoons) = 30 mL
4 fluid ounces (1/2 cup) = 125 mL
8 fluid ounces (1 cup) = 250 mL
12 fluid ounces (1 1/2 cups) = 375 mL
16 fluid ounces (2 cups) = 500 mL

WEIGHTS (mass)

1/2 ounce = 15 g
1 ounce = 30 g
3 ounces = 90 g
4 ounces = 120 g
8 ounces = 225 g
10 ounces = 285 g
12 ounces = 360 g
16 ounces = 1 pound = 450 g

DIMENSIONS

1/16 inch = 2 mm
1/8 inch = 3 mm
1/4 inch = 6 mm
1/2 inch = 1.5 cm
3/4 inch = 2 cm
1 inch = 2.5 cm

OVEN TEMPERATURES

250°F = 120°C
275°F = 140°C
300°F = 150°C
325°F = 160°C
350°F = 180°C
375°F = 190°C
400°F = 200°C
425°F = 220°C
450°F = 230°C

BAKING PAN SIZES

Utensil	Size in Inches/Quarts	Metric Volume	Size in Centimeters
Baking or Cake Pan (square or rectangular)	8×8×2	2 L	20×20×5
	9×9×2	2.5 L	23×23×5
	12×8×2	3 L	30×20×5
	13×9×2	3.5 L	33×23×5
Loaf Pan	8×4×3	1.5 L	20×10×7
	9×5×3	2 L	23×13×7
Round Layer Cake Pan	8×1½	1.2 L	20×4
	9×1½	1.5 L	23×4
Pie Plate	8×1¼	750 mL	20×3
	9×1¼	1 L	23×3
Baking Dish or Casserole	1 quart	1 L	—
	1½ quart	1.5 L	—
	2 quart	2 L	—